Diagnostic Assays for Colon Cancer

Diagnostic Assays for *Colon Cancer*

Abulkalam M. Shamsuddin, M.D., Ph. D.
Professor of Pathology
Department of Pathology
School of Medicine
The University of Maryland
Baltimore, Maryland

CRC Press
Boca Raton Ann Arbor Boston London

Library of Congress Cataloging-in-Publication Data

Shamsuddin, Abulkalam M.
  Diagnostic assays for colon cancer / Abulkalam M. Shamsuddin.
      p.   cm.
  Includes bibliographical references and index.
  ISBN 0-8493-6540-6
  1. Colon (Anatory)—Cancer—Diagnosis. 2. Tumor markers—Diagnostic use. I. Title.
  [DNLM: 1. Biological Markers. 2. Colonic Neoplasms—diagnosis. 3. Glycoconjugates—analysis.
  4. Precancerous Conditions. WI 520 S528d]
  RC280.C6S53   1991
  616.99′4347—dc20   91-19238
                                                                                                      CIP

Direct all inquiries to CRC Press, Inc., 2000 Corporate Blvd., N.W., Boca Raton, Florida, 33431.

© 1991 by CRC Press, Inc.

International Standard Book Number 0-8493-6540-6

Library of Congress Card Number 91-19238
Printed in the United States

*To the millions of fellow human beings suffering from cancer;
may this humble effort help alleviate their pain.*

THE AUTHOR

Abulkalam M. Shamsuddin, M.D., Ph.D., is Professor of Pathology at the University of Maryland School of Medicine in Baltimore.

Prof. Shamsuddin graduated from Dhaka Medical College, University of Dhaka, Bangladesh, in 1972. Following his internship and residency training, he was certified by the American Boaard of Pathology in 1977. He received his Ph. D. in Experimental Pathology in 1980 at the University of Maryland, where he had joined the faculty as an instructor in 1977, and became a professor in 1988.

Prof. Shamsuddin has been studying the process of cancer formation with an eye for practical use. By exploiting his observations in cancer markers and the histogenesis of colon cancer, he recently invented several new tests for the early diagnosis and screening of colorectal cancer, one of which has already become quite popular and is undergoing extensive study worldwide.

While he continues to strive for better diagnostic assays for cancer, he has embarked on research in cancer prevention and therapy. Prof. Shamsuddin recently discovered that the comnbined treatment of inositol, inositol hexaphosphate, and natural constituents of cereal grains such as rice, wheat, etc. effectively prevents cancer with virtually no toxic effect. While human trials are expected to be underway soon, he hopes to discern the mechanism of their action someday.

Prof. Shamsuddin has communicated the results of his research through numerous peer-reviewed papers, scientific meeting presentations, book chaopters, and invited lectures throughout the world.

PREFACE

When I was contacted by Marsha Baker to write (rather compose) a book on diagnostic assays for colon cancer, I was not sure if I could meet their expectation; a chapter or two maybe,...but a complete book!

As I started to organize my thoughts, I realized that before one embarks on using or even reading about diagnostic assays, it might be helpful to have an understanding of the background principles of such assays; and before one embarks on applying these assays for diagnosing colon cancer, it would be useful to be familiarized with the disease process itself. Having worked in this field, I cannot help but be biased toward self; I have nevertheless tried to present objective and rather balanced accounts of subject matters that are controversial. I apologize to those whose important contributions were not included. This book by no means is a replacement of the encyclopedic ones dealing with cancer, statistics, pathology, innumerable studies with occult blood tests, gastrointestinal endoscopy, or radiology. Instead, I present to you an assimilation of all these as appropriate. Apologies are also due to those who may consider it too elementary or too much in depth (unlikely); it was intentional, keeping in mind that a host of health care personnel dealing with the various aspects of colon cancer would read it. Thus, I had to balance between too much and too little.

It is almost a natural for interested health care personnel to apply the diagnostic assays in screening people for cancer. Screening a large number of people for colon cancer is however not a simple matter; thus, I have introduced this topic at the very beginning. The sequence of presentation (definitions of diagnostic and screening assays, pathogenesis of colon cancer, markers of colon cancer, current assays, new assays, and the future ones) reflects the approach I have taken towards the understanding of this subject. At the cost of being repetitious, I have stressed the importance of histogenesis of the cancer, which I think is one of the fundamental issues in studies of early marker; time and again I emphasized the field-effect of carcinogen in marker expression. In the chapter on new assays, I have tried to give a historical account of the development of the assays, anecdotes, etc., all in order to make an otherwise dry subject just a bit interesting. I sincerely hope that your expectations would be fulfilled, at least in part, by my work which I could not have done without the technical support of Perry Comegys in preparing most of the illustrations, and the moral support and encouragement from my wife Daliah and son Shomon.

A. K. M. Shamsuddin

TABLE OF CONTENTS

Chapter 3
Markers of Precancer and Cancer   **47**

Chapter 1

INTRODUCTION

I. MAGNITUDE OF THE PROBLEM OF COLON CANCER

Cancer of the colon and rectum will eventually develop in approximately 6% of the population in the U.S. and Western Europe.[1-3] It is also estimated that nearly 6 million Americans who are alive today will die of this cancer.[1] It is one of the most common cancers in the industrialized societies and the estimate by the American Cancer Society regarding its annual incidence is frighteningly increasing (over 157,000 new cases estimated for 1991).[4] As if the preceding is not bad enough, the risk of developing cancer in populations with certain diseases or family histories is even higher. Patients with ulcerative colitis and Crohn's disease of the colorectum are at very high risk of developing cancer of the organ.

Globally speaking, the incidence of colorectal cancer is generally high in populations with Western European culture and low in Africa, Asia, and South America. The highest incidence rates are reported in the U.S. (Connecticut 30.1/100,000 for colon, and Hawaiian Chinese 20.4/100,000 for rectum), New Zealand, and Scotland, and the lowest in Nigeria (1.2/ 100,000). Although data from many of the developing countries are not available, it is probably safe to assume that cancer of the colon and rectum is more prevalent in economically developed countries and more common in upper socioeconomic strata. The disease affects males and females almost equally, though a slight male predominance is seen for rectal cancer (1.2:1).

Comparisons between the Japanese in Japan vs. different generations of Japanese Americans, Jewish populations in Israel that have immigrated from Africa or Europe, or the African Americans in Alameda County in California vs. Nigerians in Ibadan (wherefrom many African Americans have originated), give important clues about colorectal cancer. While the migrants are genetically more akin to their native populations back at the origin, sooner or later, willingly or reluctantly, they adopt to the alien environment of the new home. Use of such logic and comparative analyses lead us to believe that colorectal cancer is more of a disease of our environment. Geographic epidemiology and other studies of migrant population suggest that dietary factors, particularly meat, fat, and fiber directly and indirectly influence the incidence of colorectal cancer and therefore, until today, our quest for understanding its etiology and designing strategies for prevention essentially hover around these general factors. Members of families afflicted with certain genetic diseases are predisposed for colorectal cancer, but their number is extremely small when compared to the vast majority of patients with nongenetic disease. Genetic factors are therefore considered to play a very minor role in colorectal cancer risk.

Thus, by and large, colorectal cancer is a disease of our environment (both the external and the internal environment in the colorectal lumen). Although environmental chemical carcinogens are considered to be the cause of most of our cancers, a specific carcinogen for colon and rectal cancer has not been identified. Strong DNA damaging mutagens have been identified in the feces (fecapentaenes) of high-risk individuals, but they are yet to be proven unequivocally as carcinogenic agents for the colon and rectum in experimental models, much less in humans.

II. WHY SCREEN?

While there continues to be numerous "breakthroughs" in cancer treatments, particularly in the popular news media and supermarket tabloids, the effective "silver bullet" is still in our dreams. We have yet to come up with the effective treatment for many of the cancers, and colon cancer is no exception. Effective treatment would perhaps mean cure of the disease. I am sure in the future, near or distant, we eventually will have the real breakthroughs that withstand the test of time, and cures for cancers will be found. Until that day, it is probably unrealistic to measure the success of cancer treatment with the same yardstick as that used for Strep-throat, pneumococcal pneumonia, typhoid, etc.; we have to be content with an improvement in survival rate. Carrying this point one step further, it could be argued that failure or reluctance to provide treatments which are less than cure yet increase the survival could perhaps be considered unethical. There has been progress in that direction, albeit limited, in increasing the survival rate of some cancers such as seminoma of the testis, hormone therapy of some breast and prostatic cancers, etc. For the vast majority of the cancers, including that of the colorectum, early detection and prevention is still our best hope. Not only because of this lack of therapeutic agents are we left with no choice, but it is also a matter of common sense that "an ounce of prevention is better than a pound of cure" and this applies to all our problems in life.

A. SCREENING TEST

The success of a prevention program will depend on the identification of the problem; that is the identification of people (1) with existing cancer, and those (2) who are at a risk of developing the cancer. The former (identification of people with cancer), can be done when the disease produces symptoms and the individual, now a patient, seeks medical attention. Extensive work-up including diagnostic assays are performed to identify the cancer and appropriate therapy is administered. However, regrettably that is too late for many. It identifies patients with cancer only sporadically and certainly does not prevent the cancer. Thus, to be effective, we have to have a program to actively seek individuals with cancer or high risk thereof from an apparently healthy non-complainant population. This is done by separating (or screening) individuals into groups with high and low probability of cancer of the large intestine with the help of rapid, simple, and inexpensive tests (screening tests). Implicit in the definition of the screening is a promise that there is a benefit for those who volunteer to be screened; they will be followed, with further diagnostic assays, in turn with further promise (implied) of long-term care and treatments of proven efficacy.[5]

A screening test therefore is a form of examination or a combination of examinations performed on individuals for the purpose of separating them into risk categories. These examinations could be merely questionnaire, or physical examination, X-ray, blood test, urine analysis, stool examination, Papanicolaou ("Pap") smear, sputum examination, etc. A screening test is never intended to give the full diagnosis; hence the distinction from diagnostic test. An individual that is positive with a screening test will need to undergo diagnostic procedures to confirm the presence of the disease.

B. DIAGNOSTIC ASSAY

At this juncture, it is important to point out the differences between screening and diagnostic assays and others. Diagnostic assays are applied to people who have sought health care in order to pinpoint as accurately as possible the exact cause of the sickness.[6] Aside from the individual who is obviously sick and comes for medical attention, diagnostic assays are usually done following other assays that incidentally discover a problem pointing towards cancer of the large intestine. Diagnostic procedures and assays can often be expensive, uncomfortable, complicated, time consuming, and elaborate. Incidental discovery of these problems may take place as a part of an epidemiological survey of a preselected population in the hope of obtaining new knowledge. This program is obviously initiated by an interested investigator and no promise of subsequent health benefit to the participant is implied.

A program related to disease detection is "case finding" which is quite often mistakenly referred to as screening. Case finding is a physician's incidental use of a secondary preventive maneuver for a "regular" patient during routine health check-ups for an unrelated problem. Although to be used in a mass screening program, the screening assay must meet certain rigorous criteria of net benefit to the participant (*vide infra*); it is however not so implied for "case finding".[7]

III. IDEAL SCREENING TESTS

Since the early 1960s, there have been several recommendations for cancer screening tests and programs.[8] These criteria were further developed into a uniform one by the World Health Organization (WHO) for mass screening.[9] I have taken the liberty of modifying them slightly for pertinence to colorectal cancer, the subject matter of this book. Many of you are probably familiar with the claims by various groups regarding the use of the assay of their choice for screening large intestinal cancer, such as the fecal occult blood test, barium enema X-ray, screening colonoscopy, etc. Prior to discussing them in Chapter 4, let us familiarize ourselves with the WHO criteria in order to appreciate their contributions in proper perspective.

1. Screening must lead to an improvement in end results (defined in terms of mortality, physical, social, and emotional function, pain, and satisfaction) among those in whom early diagnosis is achieved or in the other members of the community.

2. The therapy for cancer of large intestine must favorably alter its natural history, not simply by advancing the point in time at which diagnosis occurs, but by improving survival, function, or both. The modification of risk factors is not sufficient evidence of effectiveness. The measurement of survival and other end results must withstand epidemiologic and biostatistical scrutiny.

3. Available health services must be sufficient both to ensure diagnostic confirmation among those who screen positive and to provide long-term care.

4. Compliance among asymptomatic patients in whom an early diagnosis has been achieved must be at a level demonstrated to be effective in altering the natural history of large intestinal cancer (see criteria 2).

5. The long-term beneficial effects, in terms of end results, must outweigh the long-term detrimental effects of the therapeutic regimen utilized and the "labeling" of an individual as "diseased" or "at high risk".

6. The effectiveness of potential components of multiphasic screening should be demonstrated individually prior to their combination.

7. The cost-benefit and cost-effectiveness characteristics of mass screening and long-term therapy must be known. Because of the limited nature of manpower and financial resources, this information is essential in arriving at an appropriate mix of diagnostic and therapeutic services.

8. The cost, sensitivity, specificity, and acceptability of the screening test must be known and it should lend itself to the utilization patterns of the target population.

9. Ideally, an estimate of social benefit of preventing, arresting, or curing the large

intestinal cancer should be known.

10.   The appropriateness of the mix of screening tests to the target population must be considered, acknowledging that differences in the distributions of two diseases may render the combination of their respective screening tests inappropriate.

The preceding criteria (with the exception of my minor modifications), developed by the experts under the auspices of WHO, are undoubtedly the standard and the importance of each one of them can not be over-emphasized. A discussion of this issue would entail familiarity of some common terms. Following the description of these terms, we shall come back to further elaboration and discussion of these criteria in the context of colon cancer.

IV. DEFINITION OF COMMON TERMS

Some common terms used in screening, particularly with reference to colorectal cancer, are defined here. Before proceeding to define the others, I would like to bring to the attention of the readers the terminology related to the organ itself. The term "colon" as used in the title of this book refers popularly to the entire large intestine. Anatomically however, the colon is only a part of the large intestine which also includes the cecum proximally and the rectum distally. The terms "colon" or "colorectum" (as if an attempt to be more accurate) are perhaps easier to verbalize and to relate to the public and therefore has replaced the anatomically accurate but somewhat convoluted "large intestine". In the hope that this book will be read not only by the health care professionals, but also other members of the society, I have deliberately used the term "colon" in the title and interchangeably used it with colorectum and large intestine in the text. While this might cause a bit of confusion to a few, it may also serve as a reminder to the issue.

Population is the full set of individuals to whom we limit the discussion, address the issue, or make inference(s); for example, the population in the U.S., the industrialized West, industrially developing countries, etc. While our purpose is to improve the quality of life in the population (however narrow or broad), it is impossible to study the entire population. Thus, a *sample,* which is a subset of finite number from that population is taken.

Two of the most commonly used terms in the context of screening tests are sensitivity and specificity. *Sensitivity* is defined as the proportion of diseased subjects who have a positive

$$\frac{\text{Number of positives in diseased patients}}{\text{Total number of patients with disease}} \times 100$$

test. For instance, if only 70 patients out of a total of 100 with known colonic carcinoma and or precancerous lesions are positive with a screening assay, then the sensitivity of the assay is 70%. *Specificity,* on the other hand, is the proportion of nondiseased subjects who yield a negative test result. For example, in any sample, if 80 of a total of 100 otherwise normal,

$$\frac{\text{Number of negatives in nondiseased patients}}{\text{Total number of nondiseased subjects tested}} \times 100$$

disease-free individuals are tested negative with an assay, then the specificity of the assay is 80%. In general, there is an inverse relationship between the sensitivity and specificity of a test; attempts to render an assay more specific to maximize the cost effectiveness often leads to a reduced sensitivity.

Rate of positivity: expressed as the percentage of patients who have scored positive from the total screened.

$$\frac{\text{Number of patients tested positive}}{\text{Total number of patients screened}} \times 100$$

False positivity: this is the percentage of individuals that have tested positive by the screening test, but subsequent work-up revealed no pathology, hence false positive.

$$\frac{\text{Number of subjects tested positive but no pathology found}}{\text{Total number of subjects scored positive and worked up}} \times 100$$

The true rate of "false positivity" in colorectal cancer is however a difficult figure to determine. As will be noted in subsequent chapters, (1) large intestinal cancer may evolve in a manner that may be undetectable with the current technology; in other words, there could be microscopic carcinomas or precancerous lesions; and (2) the verification of whether or not there is any pathology depends on the extent of further work up. Patient follow-up is certainly an additional modality which could also be used to determine the rate of false positivity besides it being a good health care practice. The rate of false positives should be low so that unnecessary work-up is not performed on a large number of people at a considerable financial cost to the society.

False negative rate is the proportion of diseased individuals that is missed by the assay. The rate of false negative should also be low, otherwise many patients with the disease would go

$$\frac{\text{Number of diseased patients tested negative}}{\text{Total number of tested patients with disease}} \times 100$$

undetected by the assay therefore defeating the purpose at a great cost in terms of human life. A well-noted example of false negativity is that of President Ronald Reagan who was tested negative by six consecutive fecal occult blood tests, all the while harboring a cancer in his cecum.[10] It is a matter of rejoice that the President's cancer was nevertheless detected by colonoscopic examination; many fellow citizens are not so fortunate.

The *Predictive value* of a positive test is the proportion of individuals with a positive screening test who are found to have the disease as a result of further diagnostic work-up and therefore is dependent on the sensitivity, specificity, and the prevalence of the disease.

Mortality rate is the number of deaths per unit time per unit population at risk (usually expressed as per 100,000 per year).

V. COLON CANCER SCREENING

Since screening is initiated by the interested investigator and implicit in the program is a promise of some benefit to the apparently healthy otherwise normal volunteer, the evaluation of a screening program must be done very carefully and rigorously.[6] Because of this implied promise in a screening program, a greater certainty of efficacy is required when patients are solicited through screening than when patients are forced to seek medical care because of symptoms.[5,6]

The screening test should be inexpensive, safe, rapid to administer and perform, easy to apply, and, thus, must be acceptable to the population being screened. The test should have high sensitivity and specificity and good predictive value. An assay could however serve the dual purpose of being used in screening or diagnosis. The sensitivity and specificity requirements of the assay would be different depending on the use: is it for screening or is it used for diagnosis?[6] If the assay is used for diagnosis, obviously to have confidence on the assay one would like the assay to have high sensitivity; although a high specificity is desirable, it is not quite a necessity.[6] On the other hand, Prorok[6] advocates that if the assay is used for screening, the sensitivity need not be extremely high, but a reasonably high specificity is required, since low specificity can lead to an excessive number of false positive cases which could overwhelm diagnostic services, resulting in skyrocketing health care cost; That is, if you are the epidemiologist or the governmental health care administrator. The perspective would be different if you are concerned about your own health or that of your dear ones, yet do not wish to pay a high tax! The issue of false positive rate in colon cancer can be a complex one and a fruitful debate over it requires an adequate knowledge of the genesis of the cancer and the progression of the early lesions (see Chapter 2).

A. HOW TO EVALUATE A SCREENING ASSAY

Testing for unobvious bleeding in the intestine (fecal occult blood test, FOBT) has been a widely used modality to screen for colorectal cancer; other procedures have also been recommended, but the number of subjects evaluated by FOBT are far more. In recent years, there has been much debate over the cost effectiveness of screening programs for colorectal cancer using fecal occult blood test.[7,10-12]

The efficacy of a screening assay in detecting colon cancer or that of a screening program in altering the outcome of colon cancer can be evaluated by (1) experimental study, also known as randomized controlled trial, or (2) observational study, which is nonrandomized or quasi-experimental. The prevalence of cancer of the large intestine (70 to 100 per 100,000 Americans), and associated high mortality (42 per 100,000) and morbidity fulfills most of the criteria (mentioned in the Section III) to make it eligible for the benefit of screening programs. In designing the study, one must consider the following:

1. The target population should be reasonably responsive to the invitation for participation (compliance).
2. The participant should not only agree that as a result of screening, if tested positive, there would be further participation in diagnostic workup, and if cancer is discovered, the patient should undergo effective treatment, but there should also be a reasonable expectation of compliance.
3. The most important point in selecting the study population is to determine whether the participants should be symptomatic or asymptomatic, with clear criteria for such distinction.[6] Care must also be given to distinguish the population at large vs. industrial or hospital-based ones, and the assignment of individuals to screened (experimental) or unscreened (control) group should be done by randomization (or preferably stratified randomization).
4. The performance of a screening test must also be well controlled: who will do the test and who will interpret the results? What would be the training of the individuals so as to minimize the inter-individual variation of interpretation of the results?

Other factors such as co-intervention and contamination are to be addressed in the study and avoided as much as possible. Co-intervention is the performance of additional screening or other procedures on the experimental (screened) group but not on the control unscreened group. When members of the control (unscreened) group receive the test, it is contamination.

Fecal occult blood test, the prevalent assays used for screening of colon cancer has not been based on the understanding of the formation of colon cancer (see Chapter 4); newer ones are and those in the future would also be based on the expression of markers early during formation of the cancer. Thus, paramount to launching and evaluating a screening program based on these newer tests is the understanding of the natural history of colon cancer since the screening test will be detecting early or borderline lesions.[13,14] To enable you to deal with this issue, I have attempted to give accounts of the genesis of colon cancer, the precancer, and the early lesions in Chapter 2. It is of great importance that, based on the available knowledge, an agreed upon policy for classification, understanding, management, and follow-up of these early or borderline cases be established.[6,13,14]

1. Is the Detection of a Polyp Equivalent to Detection of Cancer?

Simply stated, polyps are new growths that have a variable potential to become malignant. The question then arises: should the detection of a small polyp with very negligible risk of malignant transformation be equated to the discovery of a large polyp with 50% chance of harboring a cancer? Alternatively, should the detection of even a large polyp be considered equivalent to having a cancer detected? Citing that a proportion of polyps do harbor foci of cancer, there is considerable interest among gastroenterologists to screen for and remove all the polyps in order to provide the population with a "clean colon". Given the fact that a proportion of polyps may become cancer, albeit small, it is a prudent practice to remove them once they are identified; almost like while you are in the abdomen for some other reason, why not remove the appendix lest there might be acute appendicitis at a future date. That is well justified; that is, if you are doing a colonoscopy for other indication(s) and you discover a polyp, why leave it there? But to try to justify a screening program at a cost of $450 to $750 for each colonoscopy (not to mention the discomfort associated with the procedure) to detect the polyps is another matter that will have to be debated seriously.[15]

On this issue, as regards the screening tests are we then to come up with different sets of parameters (sensitivity, specificity, predictive value, etc.), one for cancer and another for polyp? And that leads us to the end point determination which will give the outcome measurement.

2. Outcome Measurement

The outcome measure in screening for early detection and treatment of cancer will have to be the unequivocal demonstration of reduction in mortality in order to justify the cost of screening and fulfill the implied promise of benefit to otherwise healthy volunteers.[6] Thus, the end point of choice for colon cancer screening is a reduction in the mortality rate of the population. Determination of this however may take years if not decades and thus alternate short-term outcome measurements are to be looked for. One such end point measurement is the discovery of cancer, not withstanding the issue of whether or not to equate the precancerous lesions (with extremely variable risk of cancer) with cancer. Since the objective of screening for colon cancer is early detection and treatment, it would theoretically postpone death due to the cancer and therefore another alternate end point measure is the survival rate. There are however problems with using these suboptimum outcome measures, and the reader is referred to the review by Prorok.[6,16] Suffice it to say that the life expectancy of a screened population may not be substantially changed even with a successful cancer screening program; Miller asserts that for most industrially developed countries, the life expectancy would increase by a mere 2 1/2 years even if all cancers were to be eradicated.[16]

B. HOW TO MEASURE THE ACCURACY OF A SCREENING TEST

To begin with, the word "accurate" should not be used to describe either a screening test or a program.[17] One of the first points to remember in talking about screening tests is that a screening test is not diagnostic. Caution must be exercised when comparisons are made between the nondiagnostic screening test and the "gold standard" of diagnosis which is attained by biopsy, surgery, autopsy, or long-term follow-up, keeping in mind that nothing is perfect, not even the gold standard.[18]

The parameters of importance are the sensitivity, specificity, and the predictive value. There should be quality control programs to ensure that the stated levels of sensitivity and specificity are achieved and maintained.

C. HAS COLON CANCER SCREENING BEEN USEFUL?

This has been quite a debated issue for some time; in recent years, the debate seems to have intensified, perhaps initiated by the well-known case of cancer in Mr. Reagan.[7,10-12,19-21] The results of mortality and morbidity reductions due to massive screening using the FOBT are yet to come. Meanwhile, the sensitivity (not of blood in stool but of cancer or polyp), specificity, predictive values, and some estimate of cost are in. Thus far, the data have not been encouraging; the false positive rates of the FOBTs are so high that only 5 to 10% of people who screen positive actually have the disease;[19] an asymptomatic patient age 45 or older with a positive FOBT has a chance of 1 in 10 or more for having colorectal cancer![20-22] Likewise, 50 to 60% of cancers and greater than 80% of the polyps remain undetected.[19-21] The cost for detecting a cancer? Petrelli et al.[22] estimate $3825 for each cancer detected. Assuming that the annual FOBT finds 50% of the colon cancers, according to David Eddy, the annual cost for colon cancer screening for the U.S. would be approximately $1 billion.[10] Extrapolation of the cost estimates based on that by Petrelli et al.[22] (multiplying with 150,000 new colon cancer cases in the country each year), the cost to the society for detecting these new cases is $574 million. In formulating national health policy, some might consider these figures to be high, leaving the scope for the epidemiologists and politicians to debate, one must not forget the perspective from the beneficiary's end; $3825 would be a very small price for early detection of cancer with a chance for virtual cure. The important question is do we have a good screening test?[19-21,23-25]

REFERENCES

1. **Seidman, H., Mushinski, M., Gelb, S., and Silverberg, E. S.,** Probabilities of eventually developing or dying of cancer — United States, 1985, *Ca.,* 35,36, 1985.
2. **Winawer, S. J., Miller, D. G., and Sherlock, P.,** Risk and screening for colorectal cancer, *Adv. Inter. Med.,* 29, 471, 1984.
3. **Weisburger J. H., Reddy, B. S., and Joftes, D. L.,** *Colo-rectal cancer,* UICC Technical Report Series, Vol. 19, International Union Against Cancer, Geneva, 1975.
4. **Boring, C. C., Squires, T. S., and Tong, T.,** Cancer statistics 1991, *Ca.,* 41, 19, 1991.
5. **Sackett, D. L. and Holland, W. W.,** Controversy in the detection of disease, *Lancet,* August 23, 357, 1975.
6. **Prorok, P. C.,** Evaluation of screening programs for the early detection of cancer, in *Statistical Methods for Cancer Studies,* Cornell, R. G., Ed., Marcel Dekker, New York, 1984, 267.
7. **Frank, J. W.,** Occult-blood screening for colorectal carcinoma: the benefits, *Am. J. Prev. Med.,* 1(3), 3, 1985.
8. **Sackett, D.,** Periodic examination of patients at risk, in *Cancer Epidemiology and Prevention,* Schottenfeld, D., Ed., Charles C. Thomas, Springfield, IL, 1975, 437.
9. **Hilliboe, H.,** Mass health examination, *Public Health Papers 45,* World Health Organization, Geneva, 1971.
10. **Kolata, G.,** Debate over colon cancer screening, *Science,* 229, 636, 1985.
11. **Frank, J. W.,** Occult blood screening for colorectal carcinoma: the risks, *Am. J. Prev. Med.,* 1(4), 25, 1985.
12. **Frank, J. W.,** Occult blood screening for colorectal carcinoma: the yield and the cost, *Am. J. Prev. Med.,* 1(5), 18, 1985.
13. **Miller, A. B.,** Report of discussion on general principles of screening, *Screening in Cancer: A Report of UICC Workshop Toronto Canada, April 24–27, 1978,* International Union Against Cancer, Geneva, 1978, 64.
14. **Miller, A. B.,** Summary and general recommendations, *Screening in Cancer: A Report of UICC Workshop Toronto Canada, April 24–27, 1978,* International Union Against Cancer, Geneva, 1978, 334.

15. **Neuget, A. I. and Forde, K. A.,** Screening colonoscopy: has the time come?, *Am. J. Gastroenterol.,* 83, 295, 1988.
16. **Miller, A. B.,** Fundamental issues in screening, in *Cancer Epidemiology and Prevention,* Schottenfeld, D., and Fraumeni, J. F., Jr., Eds., W. B. Saunders, Philadelphia, PA, 1982, 1064.
17. **Cole, P. and Morrison, A. S.,** Basic issues in population screening for cancer, *J. Natl. Cancer Inst.,* 64, 1263, 1980.
18. Department of Clinical Epidemiology and Biostatistics, McMaster University Health Sciences Center, How to read clinical journals. II. To learn about a diagnostic test, *Can. Med. Assoc. J.,* 124, 703, 1981.
19. **Simon, J. B.,** Occult blood screening for colorectal carcinoma: a critical review, *Gastroenterology,* 80, 820, 1985.
20. **Allison, J. E., Feldman, R., and Tekawa, I. S.,** Hemoccult screening in detecting colorectal neoplasm: sensitivity, specificity, and predictive value: long-term follow-up in a large group practice setting, *Ann. Intern Med.,* 112, 328, 1990.
21. **Lieberman, D. A.,** Colon cancer screening, the dilemma of positive screening tests, *Arch. Intern., Med.,* 150, 740, 1990.
22. **Petrelli, N. J., Palmer, M., Michalek, A., Herrera, L., Mink, I., Bersani, G., and Cummings, K. M.,** Massive screening for colorectal cancer. A single institution's public commitment, *Arch. Surg.,* 125, 1049, 1990.
23. **Sampliner, R. E.,** Limitations of fecal occult blood testing, *Arch. Intern. Med.,* 150, 945, 1990.
24. **Ahlquist, D. A., Klee, G. G., and Ellefson, R. D.,** Colorectal cancer detection in practice setting, *Arch. Intern. Med.,* 150, 1041, 1990.
25. **Winawer, S. J., Schottenfeld, D., and Flehinger, B. J.,** Colorectal cancer screening, *J. Natl. Cancer Inst.,* 83, 243, 1991.

Chapter 2

APPROACHES TO THE IDEAL ASSAY

I. INTRODUCTION

The ideal assays for screening large intestinal cancer should meet certain criteria; therefore, the approach to their development should be scientific rather than empirical. Elementary to this approach is a clear understanding of the normal anatomy, histology, biochemistry, cell proliferation and cell death, and other aspects of cell biology. Once these parameters of normal are understood and well established, then we need to unravel these same parameters during the stages of cancer formation. Simple though it may sound, the roads towards understanding the normal may not necessarily be quite that easy, for one has to find the samples of the normal organ and it may be a difficult process in the human, particularly in this day and age. One must also consider an acceptable and workable definition of normal (see Section II.C).

Then comes the even more difficult process of elucidating and understanding the events taking place during cancer formation in humans. This is done with the help of experimental models, each of which has its unique limitation and contribution. Finally, the extrapolation of data from the various experimental models to the human disease ought to be done with utmost care. The following schematic diagram summarizes my approach toward this issue.

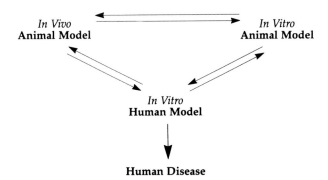

SCHEME 1. Comparison between *in vivo* and *in vitro* experimental models and with *in vitro* model of human carcinogenesis followed by extrapolation and correlation to human disease.

In the following sections, I shall try to give you an account of the knowledge gained from the experimental models only pertinent to the understanding of the genesis of the cancer as it relates to early detection. In the process, I have deliberately chosen the work of some over others, with a natural bias for my own! Likewise, in describing the human diseases, I have not attempted to make this a comprehensive text of pathology, but a brief overview of the various common lesions in order to familiarize the readers with the subject matter.

II. GENESIS OF LARGE INTESTINAL CANCER

A. MULTISTEP PROCESS OF CARCINOGENESIS

That cancer is a permanent and irreversible alteration in cellular behavior was recognized early on; the irreversibility of this new attitude of the cells readily point to an alteration in their genetic machinery. The process of cancer formation by the somatic cell mutation theory was originally proposed by Bauer in 1928.[1] This theory could explain the irreversible nature of neoplastic transformation; however, a mutational change in the genome of a cell (a rather quick process) alone can hardly explain the long latent period of cancer formation both in experimental models and in humans.[2] Subsequent experiments resulted in the theory of initiation and promotion steps of carcinogenesis[3-5] which encompass that the mutation is restricted to the first step (initiation) which is an irreversible process brought about perhaps by covalent binding of the carcinogenic agent (carcinogen) to the DNA.[6] This interaction with DNA makes cancer a genetic disease, whereby the defect in the gene of the parent cell is passed on to the daughter cells every time the cells undergo division. Initiation is irreversible in the sense that the cells with mutation may remain dormant, yet they could be activated (promoted) by promoting agents.[2-5,7-9] The irreversibility must also be looked at from the perspective of the DNA repair ability of the cell, whereby a mutational event can be repaired. Assuming that a mutation escapes repair and the cell undergoes division (with synthesis of new DNA — replication), the mutation is fixed. Cell division is therefore important for subsequent steps towards cancer development. Cancer formation currently is believed to involve complex multistep processes and interplay of numerous factors which is usually presented in simplified scheme of at least three stages, *viz.* initiation, promotion, and progression.[10-12] In as much as many models of cancer, including that of the large intestine, demonstrate these three steps, these steps may remain unobvious and often it is difficult to explain their very existence. For example, a single dose of initiating carcinogen may cause colon cancer in experimental models, the incidence of which increases with time.[13] Therefore, the proposed simple three-step carcinogenesis is a working model, one that appears to explain most, but not all, of the events during cancer formation in the colon and other organs. With further research and advancement of our understanding, in time we will revise the hypothesis again, and again…

B. EXPERIMENTAL MODELS OF LARGE INTESTINAL CARCINOGENESIS

Except for a few reports on *in vitro* models,[14-18] most of the experimental models of colon carcinogenesis have utilized *in vivo* systems. This is in part due to the difficulty in keeping the colonic epithelial cells and tissues in *in vitro* culture for a long time sufficient enough to induce and observe changes during transformation. Thus, most of our knowledge has been gained from *in vivo* models and that is what I shall discuss first.

1. *In Vivo* Models

For a detailed description of the various *in vivo* animal models, the reader is referred to the recent reviews on the subject.[19,20] I shall discuss only those aspects of the model which are directly related to an understanding of the genesis of large intestinal cancer, the subject matter of this chapter.

Most of the cancers induced in experimental animals are adenocarcinomas.[20] In the human, a benign tumor, often a precursor to cancer, called a polyp is commonly seen (*vide infra),* and experimental cancer researchers have been quick to draw an analogy between some of the induced cancers and the polyps in the human. The urge to have a paper quickly published cannot be entirely ruled out as a factor for such erroneous diagnosis since, for some time, the prevalent dogma of cancer formation in the humans had been the "polyp only-cancer theory" (implying that almost all colon cancers arise from polyps only). To state it otherwise may mean a lot of explanation with consequent delay in publication; who knows, the manuscript might never see the light of day! Suffice it to say that the vast majority of exophytic lesions of experimental animals are quite different from the benign polyps seen in humans, a fact evident to anyone who has seen them in humans as well as in animals. A few investigators have boldly pointed that out and even managed to have their papers published![21-26] Pozharisski[27]

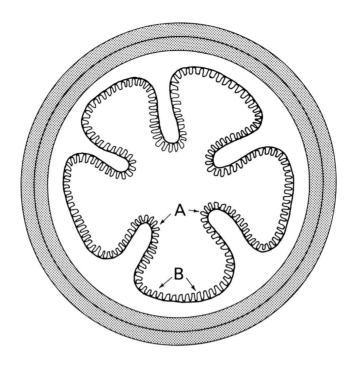

FIGURE 1. Schematic representation of the cross section of rodent colon. The rodent colon has natural mucosal folds. Neoplasms arising from the tip of the fold A are often misinterpreted as a polyp although this mucosal fold is not a true stalk as seen in human polyp (see Figure 2). An identical lesion seen in A, when situated at location B, may on the otherhand be rightly considered *de novo* cancer. (From Shamsuddin, A. K. M., Sugano, H., and

from Leningrad told us in English, rather eloquently in the *Journal of the National Cancer Institute* of the U.S.A. Alas, one could not think that he was successful, papers kept on being published claiming time and again that the experimentally induced cancers arose from "adenomatous polyps", Pozharisski could not have been a reviewer for many of those papers! Be that as it may, even a cursory examination of the published photographs of these so called "polyps" reveal that (1) they are far from human polyps, or (2) they are simply carcinomas on the tip of a normal mucosal fold, or (3) simple misdiagnosis.[27-29]

As illustrated in Figure 1, the rodent large intestine is characterized by mucosal folds that have different appearances in different segments.[30] Thus, as Pozharisski demonstrated, neoplasms arising from mucosal folds are very likely to be misinterpreted as polyps; the common pedunculated polyps in humans are composed of neoplastic "head" and apparently non-neoplastic stalk (Figure 2) and thus are completely different from the rodent exophytic neoplasms. In the humans, only a small fraction (<4%) of the common small (<1 cm in diameter) adenomatous polyps show presence of dysplastic foci that are severe enough to be called carcinoma *in situ;* if one follows some of the polyps, it may take over 15 years for a cancer to appear, that is, if it indeed does appear.[31] In contrast, in the experimental animals, those carcinomas that are not invasive from the onset, may remain in a pre-invasive stage for a relatively long time without necessarily showing dysplastic features, as seen in human polyps. In summary, contrary to the popular claims, experimental colon cancers in rodents hardly ever develop through a polyp-cancer sequence. What then is the sequence of morphogenesis?

By far, we owe it to Pozharriski[27] for his contribution to our understanding of the morphogenesis of colorectal carcinoma in an *in vivo* experimental model which is based on a rather

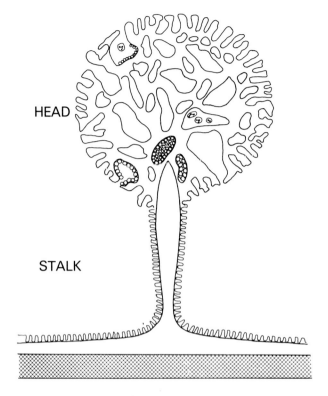

"ADENOMATOUS" POLYP

FIGURE 2.   Schematic diagram of the common pedunculated adenomatous polyp of humans which has a "drum-stick" appearance. The
neoplastic component is the head, while the stalk is composed of an
abnormal protrusion of the normal-appearing epithelium. The head is
shown to contain abnormal and dysplastic crypts. A severe degree of
dysplasia may often be called "carcinoma *in situ*". However, it is considered carcinoma when the neoplastic glands show invasion of the
muscularis mucosa (inverted V at the junction between the head and
stalk). (From Shamsuddin, A. K. M., in *Progressive Stages of Malignant
Neoplastic Growth,* Kaiser, H. E., Ed., Martinus Nijhoff, Dordrecht, The
Netherlands, Vol. 8, 1989, 64. With permission.)

extensive study on 2000 animals! The following account is a combination of Pozharriski's
work and mine.[26,27,32] The earliest changes in the colonic crypts of rodents injected with
carcinogens is an alteration in the shape of the crypts from normal, regular test tube shape[30,33]
(Figure 3) to dilated and distorted configuration (Figure 4). The crypts seem to bifurcate and
undergo branching (Figure 5). This is quite similar to the medial upheaval of the epithelial
layer at the base of the bifurcating crypts and resulting longitudinal fission as a part of the
process of increasing crypt numbers during early post-natal development.[34-36] Not only is there
an attempt to increase the number of crypts by simple fission, but the cell division is also
increased (Figure 6). These events, coupled with an increased amount of mucus production,
result in a net increase both in number and size of the glands which are by now hypercellular
(Figure 7). Not only is a polyp similar to that in the human a very rare event at best, but it is
also common not to see a high degree of atypicality or dysplasia or anaplasia in the rodents
(Figure 8). That these abnormal (although not as dysplastic as in the human) crypts are cancer
is illustrated by the elctronmicrograph of Figure 8, originally published in 1981.[26]

Taking an individual crypt as a unit, I have attempted to construct the events during

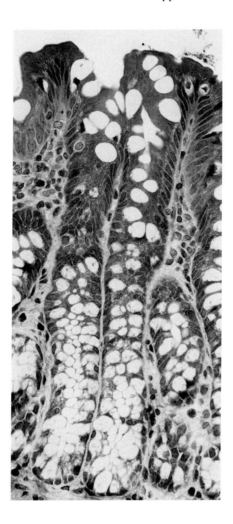

FIGURE 3. Typical test tube shaped crypts from normal rats. Similar uniform, regular crypts are also seen in the human colon when sampled at immediate autopsy, within minutes after "brain death", usually in people who die of violent trauma and free of any known disease of the large intestine; epithelia such as this serve as the standard for normal.[30]

formation of cancer in the colon and present to you my concept in Figure 9. At this juncture, I also chose to present to you Figure 10 which is to remind us all that in biology we are always confronted with the unexpected. Occasionally, one may not find any evidence of atypia, much less carcinoma or polyp in animals (including *Homo sapiens)*, yet there could be widespread metastases (Figure 10) and the colon is not the only place that you see it either. In 1973, as a resident physician in Pathology at the Baltimore City Hospitals, I had performed an autopsy on a 24-year-old patient who had widespread metastatic, poorly differentiated carcinoma and, following rather extensive search (by a compulsive resident and his even more compulsive attending pathologist Richard Slavin), the only possible source that we could find was a focus of dysplasia in his right ureter!

To summarize, in *in vivo* experimental models, following carcinogen administration, a host of changes takes place in the entire colon (diffuse yet sporadic) which show a variable degree

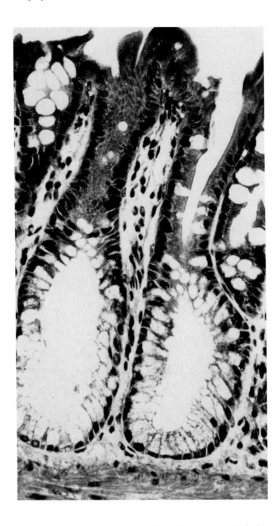

FIGURE 4. Two crypts show dilatation very early during
carcinogenesis. Compare with normal crypts in Figure 3.

of progression from normal through abnormal (precancerous) to cancer. While there are only a few recognizable carcinomas, there are many more foci of precancerous changes pointing to the fact that not all precancerous foci automatically progress to cancers and that cancer formation is a complex process. I have so far restricted the discussion on morphological changes; the other changes appropriately called markers will be discussed in Chapter 3. Suffice it to say here that carcinogenesis is a result of genomic alteration; thus phenotypic evidence of this genomic damage is likely to be expressed rather early on and perhaps throughout the entire target tissue, albeit in random foci (field effect, see Chapter 3). It appears, not unexpectedly, that of the phenotypic changes, the biochemical alterations are expressed rather early in carcinogenesis (before the formation of morphologically recognizable cancer or even dysplasia). Thus, there is a need for understanding the early events so as to be able to exploit them to our advantage in devising screening tests.

2. *In Vitro* Models

While the *in vivo* animal model has a lot to offer in terms of our understanding the pathogenesis of large intestinal carcinoma, it has its inherent limitation such as inability to do

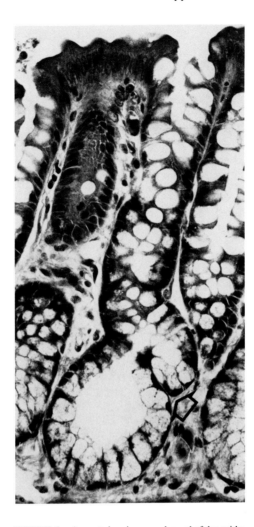

FIGURE 5.   A crypt showing an upheaval of the epithelial cells at the basal area resulting in early bifurcation (at the arrow), perhaps as a part of crypt fission[35] early during carcinogenesis.

direct experimentation with the colon epithelium and observe the resultant changes. Theoretically, *in vitro* model systems offer the solution to this limitation. In the colon, however, this has been limited by yet another factor: the inability to maintain colon for a period sufficiently long to observe carcinogen-induced changes. Most of the studies had been short-term biochemical experiments of carcinogen metabolism, carcinogen-DNA interaction, etc.[37-39] Nevertheless, the advantage of experimentation with human tissues and comparison of data with rodents *in vitro* and *in vivo* allows for a more critical extrapolation of data from animals to humans.

In general, the *in vitro* model for colon carcinogenesis has used (1) rodent colon explant culture,[17,18] (2) human colon explant culture[14,40,41] with transplantation to nude mice,[42,43] and (3) human colon epithelial cell culture.[15,44,45] In view of recent reviews by authors on these (please see References 14, 16, 38, and 39) and on tumor cell lines,[46] I shall limit the discussion germane to our understanding of carcinogenesis and their contribution in identification of new markers or concepts and relevance to screening and diagnostic assays.

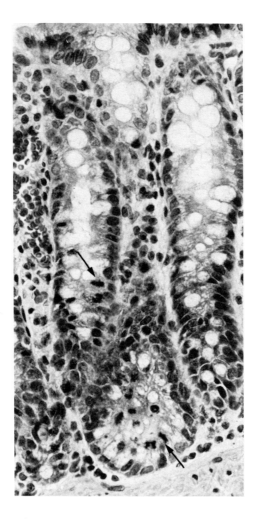

FIGURE 6.   During early stage of carcinogenesis, prior to appearance of recognizable atypical or dysplastic glands, there is increased cell proliferation as evidenced by numerous mitotic figures, only two representatives are identified with arrows; and you are challenged to identify the rest.

It is now possible to maintain human colon in explant culture for at least a month,[40,41,43] the rat colon explant may be maintained for at least 3 months, sufficient to observe carcinogen-induced early biochemical changes of mucin abnormality and morphological evidence of transformation.[17] Telang and Williams demonstrate an increase in DNA synthesis following carcinogen exposure[18] and studies in our laboratory demonstrate that following exposure to carcinogen *in vitro,* the colonic crypts are increased in number, show hypercellularity, papillary formations, and dysplasia (Figures 11 to 15). These early changes are virtually identical to those seen in the *in vivo* models, including alteration in mucin changes (see Chapter 3, Figures 3 to 7).

In the quest for maintenance of viable epithelium for a long time, Telang and Williams[18] and Valerio et al.[42] transplanted the explants to a suitable host following an initial short period of culture and maintained viable human colon tissue for at least 7 weeks.[42] Using an ingenious three-step model of carcinogen pretreatment prior to explant culture, exposure to xenotropic

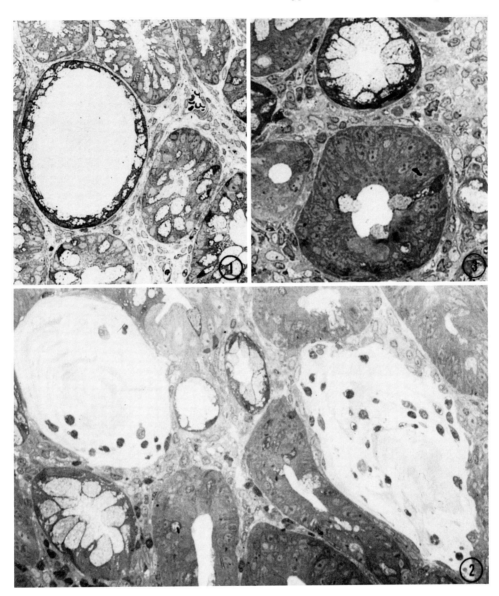

FIGURE 7. Composite of three photomicrographs in an attempt to illustrate the changes during carcinogenesis in rodents. Upper left (1) a mildly dilated crypt, bottom (2) a progressive stage of severe crypt dilatation involving two crypts that are barely recognizable as such, and finally upper right (3) an obvious neoplastic crypt with incresed cellularity, piling-up of cells, high nuclear-cytoplasmic ratio and at least one mitotic figure. (From Shamsuddin, A. M., *Arch. Pathol. Lab. Med.*, 106, 140, 1982. With permission.)

murine sarcoma virus, and then transplantation in the subcutaneous sites of athymic nude mice, Sakamoto et al.[43] have been successful in transforming the normal colon epithelium to neoplasia.

These studies[17,18,40,43] demonstrate that the colonic epithelium irrespective of its location, be it in the Petri dish or in transplanted sites in the mammary fat pad or kidney capsule, may undergo transformation if (1) a suitable carcinogen or a combination of carcinogens are used and (2) sufficient time for transformation is allowed. The preceding begs the answer to the question: why would the cancer in the human colon arise only from the polyp? Or, why could not the cancer arise anywhere in the large intestine (be in the polyp, flat nonpolyp mucosa, the bottom of a diverticulum, etc.) since the carcinogen(s) is(are) presumably in the feces?[41]

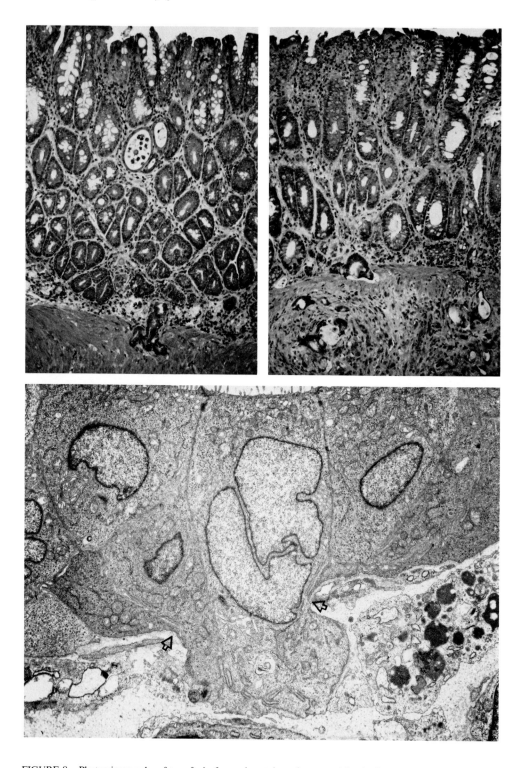

FIGURE 8.   Photomicrographs of two foci of experimental carcinomas arising in flat mucosa without polypoid excrescence (the flat mucosa and the lumen can be easily identified) are presented (upper left and right). Note that the mucosal cells show only subtle changes with conspicuous absence of dysplastic or anaplastic features, yet they are invading the muscularis layer. As mentioned in the text, it is rather common in rodent colon and not so uncommon in human colon to see lack of anaplastic feature. Electron micrographs of an intramucosal neoplastic crypt, only one to two cell layers thick, that show invasion of the basement membrane at the point between the two arrows.

STAGES IN CRYPT DILATATION

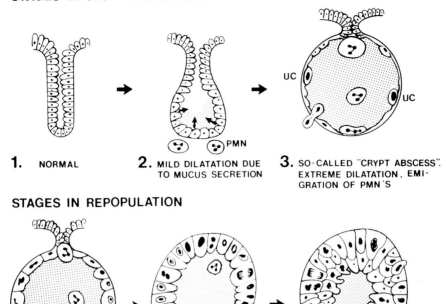

1. NORMAL
2. MILD DILATATION DUE TO MUCUS SECRETION
3. SO-CALLED "CRYPT ABSCESS". EXTREME DILATATION, EMIGRATION OF PMN'S

STAGES IN REPOPULATION

4. REGENERATION
5. HYPERCELLULARITY — MITOSIS
6. CARCINOMA

FIGURE 9.   Schematic representation of the author's concept of the stages in morphogenesis of cancer of the large intestine showing increased accumulation of mucus and polymorphonuclear leukocytes (PMN) resulting in progressive dilatation of the glands. The dilatation can be extreme, with loss of most of the lining epithelial cells (stage 3, also see Figure 7 #2); a few undifferentiated stem cells (UC) remain who undergo mitosis to repopulate the crypts. Note that with time these neoplastic cells invade the basement membrane (compare to electron micrograph in Figure 8, bottom). This may partly explain the large size of the neoplastic crypts as seen in reality in both humans and experimental models (see Figure 7 #3). (From Shamsuddin, A. K. M., Sugano, H., and Trump, B. F., *GANN Monograph in Cancer Research,* 31, 59, 1986. With permission.)

C. HUMAN DISEASE
1.   What is Normal?

For quite some time, our understanding of the normal had to depend on the use of rectal biopsy or the mucosa away from a cancer as representation of the normal large intestine. Studies in our laboratory have conclusively demonstrated how erroneous it was to extrapolate the data from those two "normal" tissues;[33,47,48] for (1) the rectum is morphologically and histochemically different from the rest of the colon, indeed the different segments of the colon are different,[33] and (2) the epithelium away from the cancer, although may look normal by the naked eye, is far from normal; indeed it shows the morphological and histochemical changes identical to the early stages of transformation in the *in vitro* and *in vivo* models. As in any scientific study, it is of paramount importance that the study of human colon also be done with appropriate and adequate controls; in this situation, the normal ought to be known. In selecting the normal as a control for comparison with abnormal, whatever the parameters may be, one must also exercise extreme care. For instance, the normal crypts of both a 30-year-old and an 80-year-old are regular test tube shaped, but those from the older individual would show a much higher rate of cell proliferation as evidenced by an increased number of mitotic figures

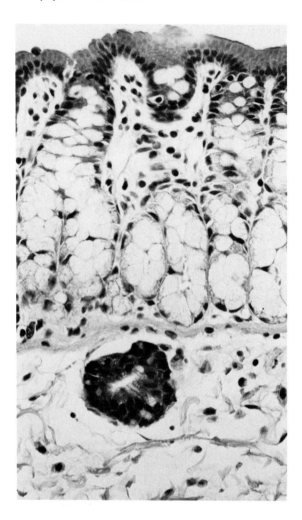

FIGURE 10. Picture to ponder! This is a photomicrograph of the colon of a rat injected with carcinogen which developed metastatic tumor. Not unexpectedly, the large intestine was free of visible cancer. In the hope of finding foci of invasive carcinoma, the entire large intestine was serially sectioned and examined under the microscope. However, no evidence of mucosal carcinoma was seen, the only abnormality being rare fission crypts (left) and cancerous glands that have already invaded beyound the *muscularis mucosa.*

than the younger counterpart (Figure 16). It is not known what causes this increased mitotic activity, but its occurrence in the elderly coincides with their higher risk of cancer; since mitosis is essential to cancer formation, a higher rate can only enhance its risk.[12]

2.   Polyp-Cancer and *De Novo* Controversy

The histogenesis of the cancer of the large intestine has been a vexingly controversial issue; it seems without much logic. There have been two views, which are so diametrically opposed that, as in political campaigns or perhaps religious convictions, often the supporters of these views have (and still would) engaged in unusually heated exchanges! Again, like political campaigns, these views were also mutually exclusive (one could not possibly be a capitalist and a communist at the same time, although such a phenomenon may now be emerging)!

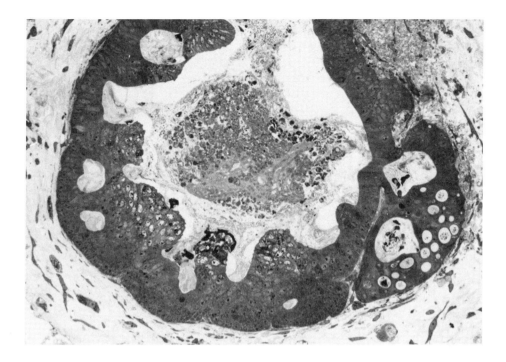

FIGURE 11. Rat colon in explant culture; one week following a single dose of carcinogen exposure, the crypts show increased cellularity, piling-up, or stratification of cells and formation of intracellular lumen.

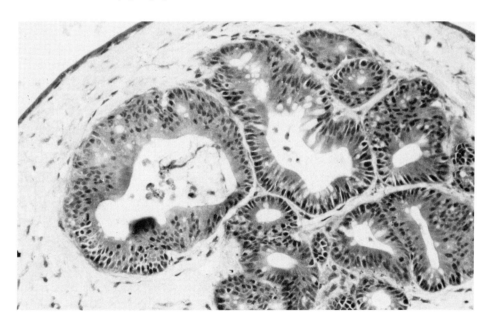

FIGURE 12. Rat colon in explant culture; two weeks following a single dose of carcinogen exposure, there is an increased number of crypts which show bizarre nuclei and focal increased cellularity, particularly in the crypts at upper left and lower right.

Subscribers of the so-called "polyp only-cancer hypothesis" believe (with deep conviction) that, except for those in ulcerative colitis, all cancers of the colon and rectum arise from preexisting polyps.[31,49] Explicit is the dogma that a cancer in the large intestine may not arise

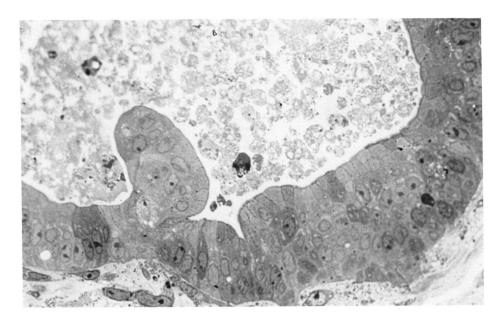

FIGURE 13. Nine weeks following a single exposure to carcinogen, the crypt shows formation of papillary projection inside the lumen, commonly seen in neoplastic glands. Note the prominent and bizarre nuclei and nucleoli.

from any place other than the polyps, thereby totally ruling out the possibility that a cancer might arise in the non-polypoid epithelium. There is no doubt that a good many polyps become cancers; somewhere between 1 and 40% polyps, depending on size, histological type, etc. harbor foci of dysplasia or cancer (*vide infra*). There is no reason not to, since polyps are also neoplasm, albeit benign. Whether or not one supports the "polyp only-cancer hypothesis", most pathologists quite often encounter cancers of the large intestine without any evidence of a preexisting polyp. Like a political battle, there are ready-made arguments to counter that: the supporters of "polyp only-cancer hypothesis" would maintain that "the polyp has been destroyed by cancer".

Perhaps one extreme draws another; the counter hypothesis calls for the development of all colorectal cancers from flat mucosa (thus, the so-called *de novo* hypothesis); they even go as far as claiming that the polyps never become malignant![50]

As a student of colon carcinogenesis, rather early in my career I was struck by the lack of logic and the degree of dogmatism in these two prevalent schools of thought. Almost simultaneously, while my laboratory experiments with the *in vivo* and *in vitro* models were progressing, I came across a case of very early yet invasive cancer in a patient. There were several foci of intraepithelial and microscopically invasive carcinomas involving in some instances only 2 to 3 crypts which, in all practicality, could not have arisen from a polyp, however small that may have been. I thought that this case would convince even the staunch supporter of the "polyp only-cancer" hypothesis that this is indeed a case of cancer arising directly from flat mucosa without going through the polyp stage (*de novo*). To make my point, I sent the histological slide of the tissue to Walter Sandritter, who at that time was the editor of *Pathology Research and Practice*. Prof. Sandritter did not take much time to publish the first report of an unequivocal case of carcinoma arising from a flat non-polypoid mucosa in the human.[51] One of the photomicrographs from that case is reproduced with permission in Figure 17. Needless to say, my enthusiasm not only to publish (from dire necessity to survive in academia!), but also to look for additional examples, paid off and over the next few years

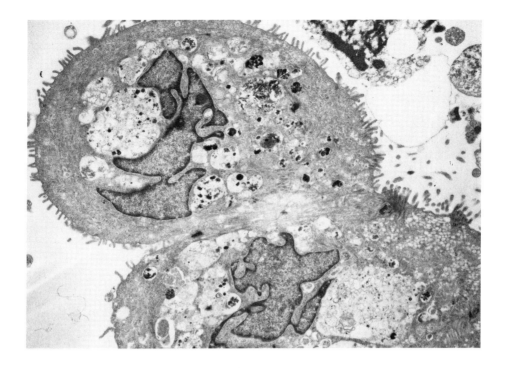

FIGURES 14. Electron micrographs of the papillary projections showing marked irregularity and invagination of the nuclear membrane.

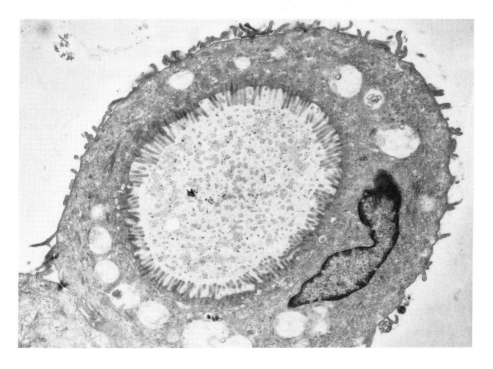

FIGURES 15. Electron micrographs of the papillary projections showing intracellular lumen with microvillar lining typical of adenocarcinomas.

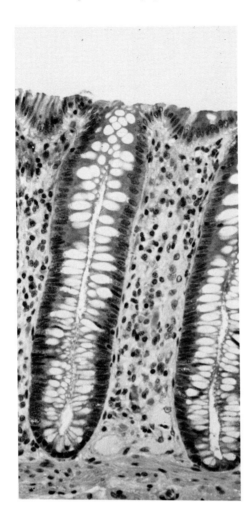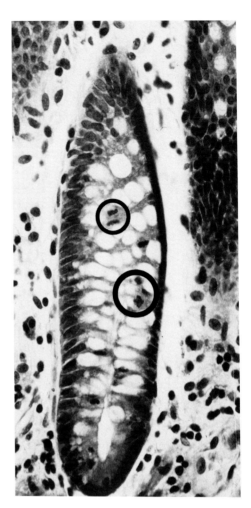

FIGURE 16. Normal colonic epithelium in a young (left) and an 84-year-old individual (right). Note the conspicuous presence of mitotic figures in the elderly.

I reported additional cases.[52-54] By this time, others have also started to report unequivocal cases,[55] but I have taken the wrath of opponents who decried that my "articles are dangerous and represent a threat to both the health of patients and the credibility of diagnostic pathologists!"[56] It is now, however, becoming increasingly evident that a good many cancers of the large intestine do not arise through the polyp stage. In a study of 951 cases (having 123 early lesions and 853 advanced cancers) of colorectal carcinomas, Shimoda et al.[57] identified lesions that were either polypoid carcinomas or nonpolypoid carcinomas without intramucosal protuberant growth. Following extensive histopathological examination, the authors conclude that nonpolypoid early carcinomas progress rather easily to advanced carcinomas and that carcinomas arising *de novo* comprise 78.2% of total cancers of the large intestine! Note that only about 17 years ago Muto et al.[31] claimed in the same journal (*Cancer*) that most of the cancers arise through the polyps only! As if the preceding is not a strong enough argument, from a study of 323 patients with adenomatous polyp, Lotfi et al.[58] report that subsequent metachronous colorectal carcinoma developed in 6.2% of the patients, but most often at sites different from that of the previous polyp!

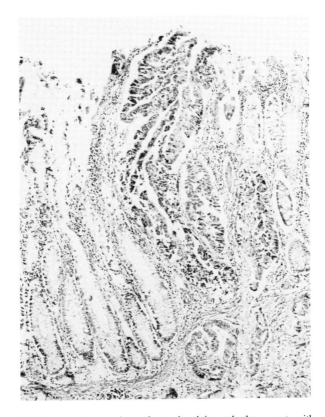

FIGURE 17. Microscopic carcinoma involving only three crypts with invasion beyound the *mucularis mucosa* is shown in a human. (From Shamsuddin, A. K. M., Bell, H. G., Petrucci, J. V., and Trump, B. F., *Pathol. Res. Pract.*, 167, 374, 1980. With permission.)

D. UNIFIED CONCEPT OF GENESIS

Be that as it may, in a short paper reporting two cases of microscopic neoplasia, I first proposed a unified hypothesis that the cancer in the large intestine arises both from the polyps and the flat mucosa *de novo*.[53] Not unexpectedly, it had provoked unkind comments.[56] I had argued, as I still do, that it is the epithelial cells in the crypts of the colon that are the precursors of carcinoma. As the *in vitro* experiments show, these cells can be transformed with proper carcinogenic stimuli even if they are in the Petri dish, or in another animal.[17,18,43] Thus, there is no logical reason as to why only the polyp will become cancer and the epithelial cells in the flat nonpolypoid mucosa will not undergo neoplastic transformation. Since the adenomatous or the villous polyps (*vide infra*) are already neoplastic in nature with abnormal cell proliferation of the crypts,[49] it is only natural to expect that they are likely (perhaps more so) to undergo neoplastic transformation. Not only is the flat nonpolypoid mucosa susceptible to malignant transformation, but also in the diverticulum or amebic and tubercular lesions.[53,59-61] It would not be illogical to think that fecal carcinogen such as fecapentaene[41] could be the initiator and that the nonspecific injuries such as amebiasis, tuberculosis, or other long-standing irritant directly or indirectly act as promoters, resulting in obviously increased cell proliferation[8,11,12] and even more obvious cancer. This point will be stressed again in the subsequent sections. What factor or combination of factors result in progression of the polyps to cancer is unknown, much less what causes the polyps to appear in the first place.

III. HUMAN PATHOLOGY

A. PRECANCEROUS CONDITIONS AND LESIONS

There are some disease conditions such as inflammatory bowel diseases of the large intestine, which with time and severity could result in cancer formation in the organ. The mere presence of these diseases however does not imply that a cancer is imminent. However, the patient is at a higher risk than the population at large.[62] The large intestine of these patients may, in the course of time, develop lesions that can be morphologically recognized by the pathologist as a part of the spectrum in the formation of cancer (precancerous lesions). These changes include variable and progressive stages of derangement of the normal histology of the epithelium towards cancer. Besides these changes (dysplasia or atypia), cancer formation in the large intestine may also take place in a preexisting polyp. Cancer formation in the large intestine, as mentioned before, may however take place directly in an otherwise normal-appearing epithelium, in the absence of any of these conditions and lesions.[51-55,57] It is to be emphasized here that while these known conditions and lesions do pose an increased risk of cancer, cancer by no means is an eventuality. In other words, not all patients with polyps or inflammatory bowel disease, etc. will develop cancer, inasmuch as not all patients with dysplasia of the uterine cervix will get an invasive carcinoma of that organ.

1. Polyps

What are these polyps that are the center of such controversy? Polyps are abnormal protrusions in the lumen of the gastrointestinal tract which could be neoplastic, hyperplastic, inflammatory, or hamartomatous in nature. The inflammatory and hamartomatous polyps (juvenile polyps and Peutz-Jeghers polyps) are rather uncommon. Perhaps because of their rarity and lack of interest to doggedly investigate them, they are not documented to pose an increased risk of cancer; and they are not immune from developing cancer either, as evidenced by several case reports documenting cancer formation at long-term clinical follow-up.[63-66]

The most common (90%) polyps are the hyperplastic polyps which are usually seen in the recto-sigmoid areas of the intestine; the neoplastic polyps are second most frequent. The hyperplastic polyps are also called metaplastic polyps and are seen in nearly 75% of people over the age of 40 years.[67] The prevalent opinion of most has been that these common, tiny (usually 1 to 5 mm in diameter) lesions are incapable of progressing to cancer and therefore are not precancerous. Once again, that is only the dogma; cancer has been reported to arise from these polyps[68] and even more interestingly, these polyps express markers identical to the cancer,[69-73] and they themselves may often be the sentinel marker of the carcinoma elsewhere in the intestine.[74]

The polyp that has gained the most fame in the literature is called adenomatous polyp which on naked eye examination may be either pedunculated or sessile or combination of both (see Figure 18). Microscopically, the neoplastic component (head) may show either tubular glands (most common), or finger-like projections (villous), or a mixture of both, hence called tubulovillous.[31] A spectrum of changes ranging from mild dysplasia to invasive carcinoma can be observed in polyps (Figure 19), the diagnosis of carcinoma being reserved for only those cases with definite invasion of the muscularis mucosa. Is the prevalence of cancer the same for all the polyps?...No. The adenomatous polyps that are most common are smaller than 1 cm in diameter and have a very low prevalence of malignant foci (1%), while the prevalence of malignant foci increases with the size of the polyp.[31] The less common villous polyps (Figure 20) are more often associated with foci of cancer in them.[31] There are some rare polyps which show a mixture of adenomatous and hyperplastic features and they are so named.[75]

The adenomatous polyps are distributed throughout the large intestine with some variation between different study populations. The distribution of the polyps, when similar to that of the carcinoma, has been used by the proponents of the "polyp-only cancer" hypothesis in favor of their argument and certainly the association is interesting. In more practical terms, while

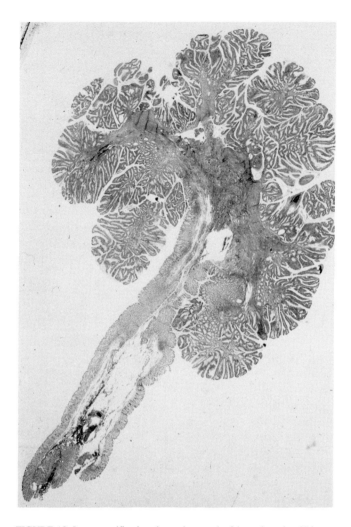

FIGURE 18. Low magnification photomicrograph of the pedunculated "drum-stick"-shaped polyp showing the neoplastic head and non-neoplastic stalk.

using diagnostic and/or screening assays, we have to be cognizant of the fact that these precancerous polyps may also occur in the right colon. As discussed in Chapter 4, there has been a tendency to advocate use of the sigmoidoscope for screening colorectal cancer which is likely to miss at least half of the polyps that may be located in the transverse and right colon combined.[76]

2. Inflammatory Bowel Diseases

The inflammatory bowel diseases (IBD) are a group of idiopathic disorders which include ulcerative colitis and Crohn's disease. There may be some overlap in terms of the morphological presentation of the two diseases and the term "colitis indeterminate" is coined for those not so uncommon situations. Ulcerative colitis (UC) can be seen in infancy and childhood, but presents most often between the second and fifth decade. The disease is more common in whites than blacks; and of the whites, it is most commonly seen in Jewish populations. Patients with UC are at a high risk of developing cancer of the large intestine, proportionate to the extent of the disease at diagnosis. The age at diagnosis appears to be an important variable, those less than 15 years have the highest risk, and the longer the duration of the disease, the higher is the risk.[77,78]

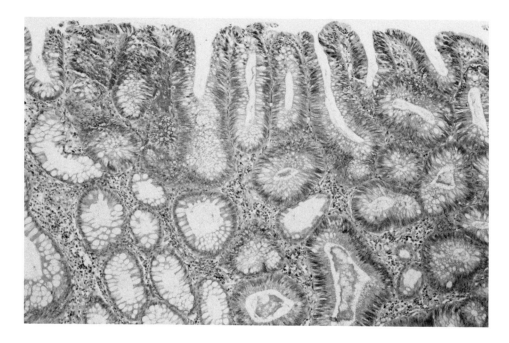

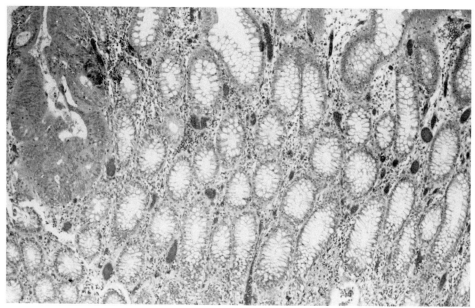

FIGURE 19. Common histological appearances of the neoplastic polyps: top — focus of mild dysplasia (lower right) in an adenomatous polyp, bottom — carcinoma *in situ* (upper left) in an adenomatous polyp.

There is mucosal inflammation, ulceration, dilated crypts containing neutrophils (so-called crypt abscess), and regeneration of crypt cells. The latter results in an accelerated rate of loss of crypt cells (normal turnover time for most of crypts cells is 72 h), resulting in fewer mature goblet cells replaced by mostly basophilic regenerated epithelial cells (Figure 21). Note the striking similarity with the early changes of *in vivo* experimental model of carcinogenesis (Figures 7 and 9). Could the two processes (ulcerative colitis and carcinogen-induced cancer in rodents) be the same accelerated models of the cancer in humans?

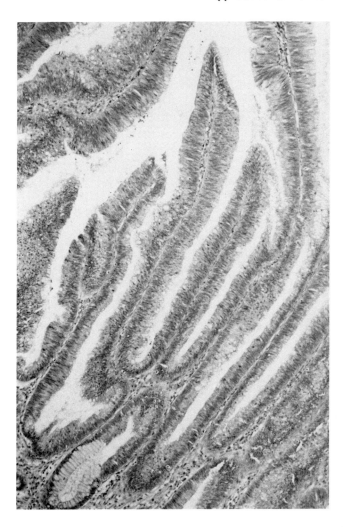

FIGURE 20. Villous polyp with finger like projections towards the lumen (compare with the test tube shaped glands of adenomatous polyps in Figure 19).

It is rather curious that although the increased susceptibility and incidence of dysplastic changes (precancerous) and cancer in the large intestine of patients with ulcerative colitis has received quick acceptance by both pathologists and clinicians alike. That a similar phenomenon could also be at play in cases of Crohn's disease of the colon was received rather coldly. Following Jones's publication in 1969,[79] several investigators have subsequently demonstrated an increased incidence of cancer in the colon affected with Crohn's disease.[80-82] Most recently, from a study of 1655 patients with Crohn's disease, Ekbom et al.[83] report a relative risk of colorectal cancer for Crohn's disease of the colon to be 5.6; those patients who are diagnosed before age 30 with any colonic involvement have a relative risk of 20.9.

In light of my experimental observations and rather simple logic, I could not see any reason why one would not expect to find precancerous changes in the colons affected with Crohn's disease. Robert Phillips, then a sophomore medical student at the University of Maryland came to me for a research project and you can guess what it was! Rob and I did find a spectrum of changes, some of which were subtle dilatation and distortion of the crypts, yet resembling the early changes seen in *in vivo* experimental models and in human colon remote from cancer. We also found classical histopathological features of dysplasia.[84] Unfortunately, this report

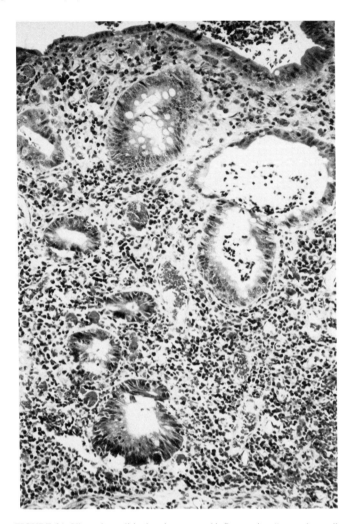

FIGURE 21. Ulcerative colitis showing mucosal inflammation, "crypt abscess", preponderance of basophilic cells, and sparse mature goblet cells (note the similarity with the experimental model, Figures 7 and 9). A crypt showing dysplastic features is seen at the bottom.

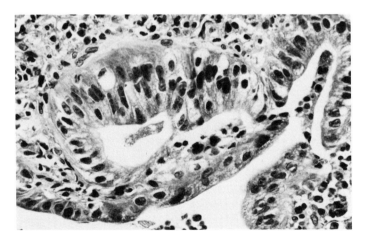

FIGURE 22. Dysplasia in Crohn's disease. (From Shamsuddin, A. K. M. and Phillips, R. M., *Arch. Pathol. Lab. Med.*, 105, 283, 1981. With permission.)

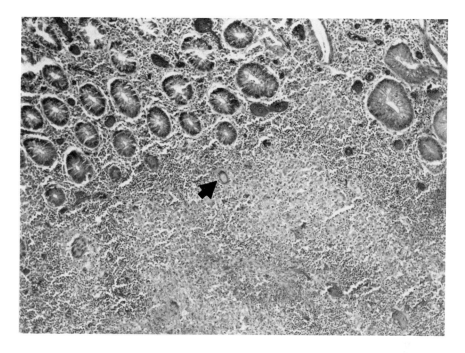

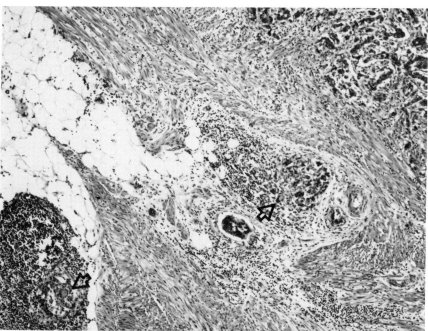

FIGURE 23. Crohn's colitis showing granulomatous inflammation (top). A giant cell (arrow) can be seen in the center. Adenocarcinoma arising in the intestine affected with Crohn's disease (bottom). The chronic granulomatous inflammation with giant cell (center and lower left field (arrows) is seen adjacent to the infiltrating adenocarcinoma.

also had drawn some not so kind response from members of the Inflammatory Bowel Disease-Dysplasia Morphology Study Group.[85] Our explanation, on a scientific premise such as in the context of initiation, promotion, and progression,[86] however must have been convincing; subsequent reports of dysplasia in the colonic epithelium in inflammatory bowel diseases (including Crohn's disease) illustrated dysplastic crypts virtually identical to those we had reported.[84,87] So that you are not distracted by these common academic squabbles, let me reiterate that any condition that would enhance cell proliferation would therefore be likely to enhance cancer formation in the large intestine (Figures 22 and 23); for that matter, in any organ.[9,12]

3. Other "Nonspecific" Injuries and Conditions

An increased proliferation of epithelial cells and resultant increase in cancer in the large intestinal epithelium can be induced by a host of factors such as diverticular disease with or without inflammation,[59,88] colostomy,[89,90] anastomoses (e.g., post-resection anastomosis,[91,92] and uretero-sigmoidostomy[93-96]), foreign body granuloma,[8] bacterial or fungal infection,[9,61] parasitic infestation,[60,97] etc. both in experimental models and in humans, almost perfectly befitting the initiation and promotion stages of carcinogenesis seen in all other organs.[9] In some of these human diseases, not only is there increased cell proliferation and dysplastic features, but the qualitative changes in mucin during carcinogenesis have also been documented by histochemical techniques.[98]

In this context, it is important to point out another common misnomer, if not a misconception, which is the so called "recurrent" cancer. This lax use of the term is not only scientifically wrong but may also open the door for unnecessary litigation. At the time of surgical resection of the colorectum for cancer, the pathologist routinely checks for the presence (rather, documentation of the absence) of cancer at the resection margin. Thus, in the vast majority of cases when the resection margin is free of cancer, from where does the recurrent carcinoma arise? Could it be implantation of tumor cells at the resection margin as some suggest? This is difficult, if not impossible, to prove and, given the skill of the surgeon and the precautions routinely taken, this alone cannot explain the high incidence of the so-called recurrent cancer at the anastomotic sites. Based on the field effect theory that I have proposed[47,48] (see Chapter 3 for detail), combined with the initiation, promotion, and increased cell proliferation, I offer the following:

1. In a patient who has a cancer of the large intestine, the entire field of the large intestine is exposed to initiating carcinogen which caused genomic changes in multiple sites throughout the epithelium.
2. Only one or two of these sites have been promoted (perhaps by bile and others) to cancer. The normal-appearing epithelium, however, demonstrates other phenotypic alterations secondary to the genotoxic damage during initiation. It does this in the form of mucin histochemical change and the expression of other markers (see Chapter 3). One of these mucin changes is expression of sialomucin instead of the normal sulfomucin; the former may be seen as far as the resection margins of the colonic segment removed for cancer![47,48]
3. Anastomosis of the resected margins requires suturing, which increases cell proliferation[8] and therefore now promotes the initiated, previously dormant, cells to cancer which is most commonly seen in the anastomotic sites.[91,92]

Support for such an explanation is beginning to emerge from data by other groups showing abnormal DNA ploidy in mucosa remote from carcinoma[99] and abnormal cell proliferation kinetics,[100-102] among others, as discussed in Chapter 3. The emergence of such a marker as a definite indicator of initiation that, when promoted, leads to increased cancer, is supported by the work of Dawson et al.[103] The development of these new cancers, which should be appropriately called "metachronous lesions", is correlated ($p < 0.0001$) with the appearance of abnormal sialomucin at either of the surgically resected margins of the original specimen.[103]

Aside from the sporadic cancers, acquired perhaps due to environmental carcinogens, members of certain families are afflicted with an unusually high incidence of carcinoma of the colon, secondary to genetic predisposition. Several such familial conditions have been described; for example, Familial Polyposis Coli, Gardner syndrome, Turcot syndrome, etc. Patients with these conditions acquire multiple adenomatous polyps, and by the third decade, most have cancer. These people are not to be screened but should be under rigorous surveillance.

B. CARCINOMA

Fully developed carcinomas of the large intestine are either cauliflower-like exophytic (common in cecum and ascending colon) or of the infiltrative and ulcerating type (most often in the distal large intestine). It is quite possible that the exophytic types may arise predominantly from the polyps and the infiltrative ones *de novo* from the flat nonpolypoid epithelium.[53] The infiltrative type usually extends through much of the circumference of the intestine, resulting in "napkin ring" deformity with a central narrow opening. An obvious complication is obstruction; a somewhat brighter side of this dismal condition of luminal narrowing is the "apple core" appearance in the barium enema picture, allowing the radiologist to make the diagnosis (see Chapter 4, Figure 11).

Irrespective of the naked eye appearance, microscopically the vast majority of the carcinomas are composed of glandular elements which are recognized, more or less, as such (well, moderate or poorly differentiated; see Figure 24). Within the same tumor, there could be areas of well-formed glands as well as complete anaplasia.

The glandular carcinomas produce a variable amount of mucin (Figure 25). Arbitrarily, pathologists reserve the diagnosis of mucinous (or colloid) carcinoma for those neoplasms where greater than 50% of the neoplasia is mucinous.[104] The natural incidence of mucinous carcinomas in the elderly is 5 to 15% of the total carcinomas.[105,106] However, in adolescents,[107,108] patients with ulcerative colitis,[106] or patients following radiation,[109] the predominant histology is that of mucinous carcinoma. Interestingly, while the experimental animals induced with chemical carcinogens also have a low incidence of mucinous carcinomas, those irradiated with X-ray show a high incidence of mucinous carcinoma.[110] The mucinous carcinomas offer a poorer prognosis than the glandular carcinoma. A variant of mucinous carcinoma called "signet ring" carcinoma (intracellular mucin) is associated with even poorer prognosis. There are other rare histological types such as squamous, adenosquamous, basaloid, small cell, etc. However, the prognosis of the vast majority of carcinomas depends, in large part, on the extent of the disease; that is, degree of penetration of the wall and spread to metastatic sites.

The popular Dukes classification,[111] which has undergone modifications,[112] and the new TNM[113] systems are most often used for estimating the severity of the disease and hence the prognosis. The original Dukes classification is as follows:

A.   The cancer has spread by direct continuity into the submucosa or muscle (but not beyond). There is no lymph node involvement.
B.   The cancer has spread beyond the muscle layers into the serosa and pericolic or perirectal tissues, but no lymph node involvement.
C.   The cancer has spread to the lymph nodes.

The 5-year survival rate, a standard way of expressing the prognosis of a cancer patient, is approximately 100% for Dukes A, 50 to 65% for Dukes B, and 20 to 40% for Dukes C. The prognosis is much worse for metastases to distal sites, commonly the liver (Dukes D).

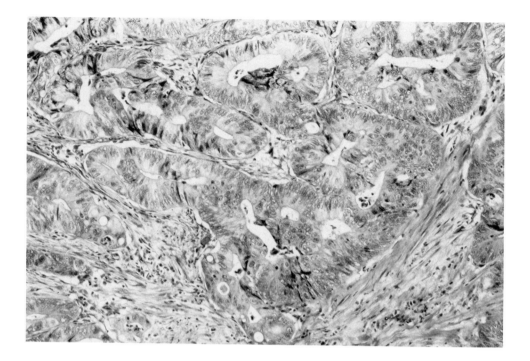

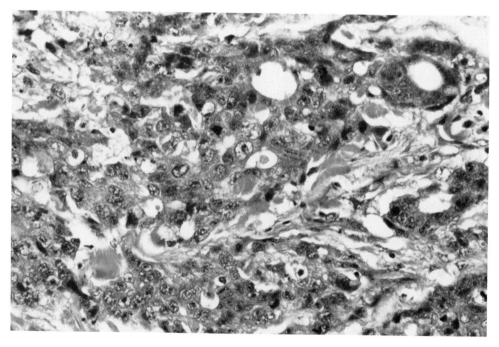

FIGURE 24. Glandular adenocarcinoma: well-formed glands can be easily recognized (well differentiated) (top); glandular structures are poorly formed, yet they can still be recognized as such (moderately differentiated) (bottom); poorly differentiated adenocarcinoma showing very little or no recognizable glandular architecture (opposite). These designations are highly subjective with marked interpathologists variations, one pathologist's moderately "differentiated neoplasm" could be another's "poorly differentiated".

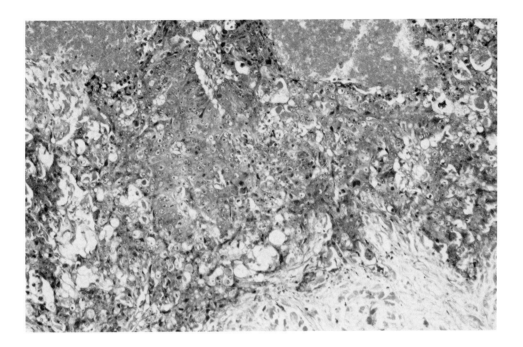

IV. REQUIREMENTS OF AN IDEAL SCREENING ASSAY FOR COLON CANCER

I have discussed in Chapter 1 the requirements of an ideal screening assay in so far as the cost-benefit to the society. In the following discussion, there will be some deliberate repetition in order to point out the areas that are pertinent to colorectal cancer. I shall, however, try to restrict my comments in context to the benefit the patient is expected to derive; in other words, who are at risk and who should be screened? At what age should we start screening the population? Who are at high risk of cancer and when should one start screening them? What should be the extent of diagnostic work-up; for example, sigmoidoscopy or total colonoscopy? What is the end point measurement of the success of the screening program; if polyps are diagnosed and removed, is that to be considered satisfactory, etc.? Let us consider these issues in some order of priority.

A. GOALS FOR COLON CANCER SCREENING

As in any other disease, the objective of the screening program for colorectal cancer must be defined. As proposed by Cole and Morrison,[114] the following could be the objectives: application of a relatively simple, inexpensive test to a large number of persons in order to classify them as likely or unlikely to have colon cancer to reduce its associated mortality and morbidity at a reasonable cost to the program. Elimination of death from colorectal cancer is not considered to be a realistic goal for screening programs since there are inherent limitations of the screening tests and programs.[114]

B. WHO IS TO BE SCREENED?

Obviously, the population at risk is to be screened. However, a screening program will invariably attract people who have signs and symptoms of colorectal cancer (thanks to the public awareness from the mass media). These patients are not to be included in a screening program since that is beyond the scope of screening activity.[114] In order to determine the sensitivity and specificity of the assays, investigators however erroneously resort to inappro-

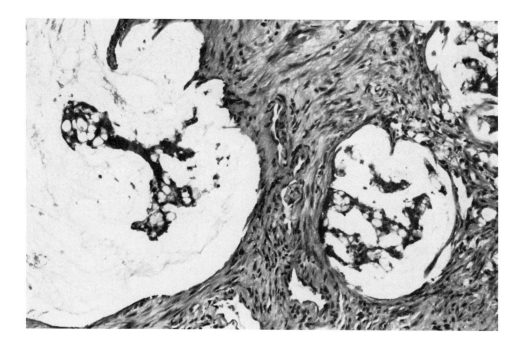

FIGURE 25A. Mucinous adenocarcinoma: colloid carcinoma showing neoplastic cells with intracellular mucin that are in "lakes" of extracellular mucin (clear spaces). Note that the neoplastic cells lining the mucous "lake" lack the general features of malignancy.

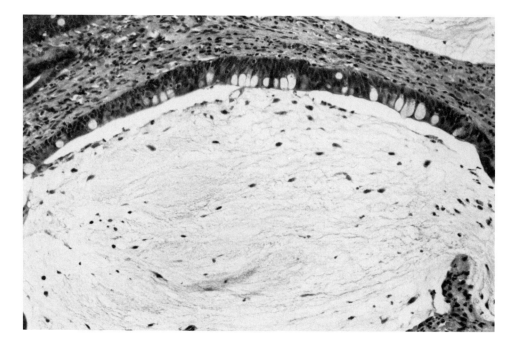

FIGURE 25B. An otherwise well differentiated glandular adenocarcinoma that contains large areas of mucinous components.

priate measures. A common error is to test a group of patients hospitalized for colorectal cancer or go to an endoscopy clinic to look for patients that are suspected of having cancer or polyp. This is a basic flaw in the study since patients with manifest clinical disease are beyond the preclinical phase and are not to be screened.[114,115] If the screening test is done on such selected patients and then used in a population of asymptomatic persons, the sensitivity is likely to be lower than the estimate based on patient population with colon cancer. The sensitivity of a particular screening test is estimated if follow-up diagnostic assays (including the histopathological diagnosis) are performed to screen both negative and positive individuals.[114] It is however impractical and perhaps unethical to subject thousands of screen negative, otherwise normal healthy people to complete colonoscopy and biopsy. At a rate of at least $4000 for diagnostic work-up for each cancer detected,[116] one cannot expect such reimbursement for normal healthy people. Besides the discomfort and the risks, however little it may be, it also cannot be justified. How then can we estimate the sensitivity and specificity of a given test? The usual and acceptable approach is a follow-up of screen negative persons to find out how many of them eventually develop cancer, the duration and thoroughness of which will certainly influence the estimate of sensitivity.[114] A yearly follow-up is the recommended frequency.[116]

Another common flaw in the study design for evaluating the efficacy of a particular screening test is the comparison of two screening tests with each other. If the principles of the two tests are different, one detects an earlier form of cancer than the other, then the tests are being evaluated against different standards and their apparent sensitivities are not to be compared.[114] This is, however, a temptation which cannot be resisted by most; the governmental regulatory agencies expect it, and the manufacturers of the assay would like to comply with the wishes of the government regulators and point to the public and health care professionals that the newer test is just as good as the old one, if not better and so on.

There are different definitions of sensitivity too; it must be clearly defined before jumping to conclusions. What is it for? Is it for cancer? Is it for precancer? Or, is it for something else? For example, one would like to think that the sensitivity of fecal occult blood test (FOBT) would be for cancer; but in real terms, its sensitivity is for detection of blood which may or may not be (most often, not) associated with cancer! Thus, when compared to ^{51}Cr-labeled red blood assay, the FOBTs have a rather high (~95%) sensitivity; alas, it is several fold less than that for cancers and even lower for precancers or polyps.[117]

An issue that is often overlooked is the reliability of the screening test, which is the ability of the test to reproducibly give the same result on repeat examination of the same subjects within a reasonable time (days or weeks). A common misconception surrounding the performance of a test is the assignment of the term "nonspecificity" to a test that detects two or more diseases, albeit a positive attribute of a test.[114] If a given test can indeed detect more than one disease, then it is even better. For instance, Cole and Morrison[114] argue that it is the strength and not limitation of the carcinoembryonic antigen (CEA) assay that it detects breast cancer as well as colon cancer; the real limitation of CEA is its false positive reactivity in disease-free individuals.

Let us come back to the question as to who is to be screened. That seems to be easy to answer: asymptomatic individuals at high risk. Those who are at high risk and are symptomatic, such as patients with inflammatory bowel diseases, persons with a personal history of prior cancer or polyp, or those with a family history of cancer, etc., are not to be screened; they are to be closely monitored.[115]

C. IS COLORECTAL CANCER A CANDIDATE FOR A SCREENING PROGRAM?

For colorectal cancer to be eligible for a cost-effective screening program, the following criteria are to be met: (1) it must have serious consequences and be so recognized by members of the target population; the high mortality rate (42 per 100,000) of the disease makes it eligible on that basis; (2) a disease must have treatment since it would be unreasonable to screen for, if it cannot be treated. There appears to be some improvement in survival following treatment of colorectal cancer. (3) To justify the cost-effectiveness of a screening program, the preclinical phase of the disease should have high prevalence. The issue becomes complicated for colon cancer, particularly in relation to genesis.

D. PREVALENCE OF POLYP VS. PREVALENCE OF CANCER: DO THEY MATCH UP?

The prevalence of the polyps "that matter" (i.e., the adenomatous polyps) has been reported to be between 0 and 69% depending on the study design and study population,[104] most data suggest that over 60 years of age, 1 in 4 people have the polyp; the prevalence gradually increased with higher age. There are two important questions: (1) what percentage of these polyps become cancer? and (2) what percentage of cancers come from polyp? There is a tendency to mix the two issues.

Based on the study by Muto et al.,[31] which is used in most modern day arguments on the relationship between polyps and cancer, 60% of the polyps are less than 1 cm in diameter and 1.3% of these are associated with cancer; 23% are 1 to 2 cm and 9.5% contain foci of cancer, while the remaining 17% are greater than 2 cm in diameter, 46% of which may contain cancer. Assuming there are 100 patients, each with 1 polyp, there will be

- 0.78 (1.3% of 60) cancers in the 60 patients with <1-cm polyps
- 2.18 (9.5% of 23) cancers in the 23 patients with 1- to 2-cm polyps
- 7.8 (46% of 17) cancers in the remaining 17 patients.

Thus, a total of 10.78 cancers should be present in the 100 polyp-bearing individuals. The result of the 1990 U.S. census is yet to come; that of 1980 shows ~15% (or 1/7) of the population to be greater than 60 years age. Assuming that the prevalence rate of the polyp in the greater than 60-years age group is 1 in 4, the prevalence rate for the entire population should be 1 in $4 \times 7 = 1/28$. Therefore, according to the rate of polyp-cancer association by Muto et al.,[31] the calculated prevalence of the cancer in the U.S. should be

$$\frac{10.78 \times 100}{28} = 0.385\%$$

In other words, the expected prevalence of cancer in the U.S. should be 385 per 100,000. Both the IARC (International Agency for Research in Cancer) and UICC (International Union Against Cancer) estimate the prevalence for cancer of the large intestine in the U.S. to be approximately 72 per 100,000.[118,119] This is a 5.3-fold lower prevalence than 385 per 100,000 expected from the study of Muto et al.[31]

This simple calculation shows how complex the issue is and that there is little room for dogmatism. Even if none of the cancers arise from flat mucosa without going through polyps (according to Shimoda et al.[57] 78% arise from the flat mucosa!), the expected and observed prevalence rates are too far apart. One must therefore look at these issues rather critically, putting aside individual biases.

This issue is more than academic; let us consider the following: assuming that almost all the cancers of the colon arise from the polyps, simple removal by an endoscopist should result in a colon cancer-free world in a rather short time. We would however live with a false sense of security if indeed even 1% of the cancers arise from the flat mucosa without going via the polyp. The vast majority of polyps detected during a screening colonoscopy, for instance, are most likely to pose very little threat to the patient's health; they have little potential for malignancy. Thus, equating the detection of cancer with that of the polyp cannot be logical.[120]

If indeed 78% of the cancers do arise without going through the polyps,[57] it poses an enormous challenge to us, the health care professionals, in terms of detection of the cancer at an early stage. While polyps are easily visible by endoscopy and removed, for microscopic cancers involving only a few crypts that more readily invade,[51,57] detection of early lesions may not be so easy. It would require both the endoscopist and the pathologist to be cognizant, and acceptance of these very facts can be rewarding.[54]

E. OUTCOME MEASUREMENT

The outcome of the diagnostic assay following screening for cancer of the colon is obviously cancer. But what about a scenario which I predict would be rather common, such as this: the result of the screening test is positive, the individual has undergone extensive diagnostic work-up (including colonoscopy at considerable cost) and discomfort, and the report is negative; in other words, the endoscopist could not find a lesion suspicious enough to biopsy. In another extreme example, a biopsy is done and is read negative by the pathologist. Can the individual rest assured that there is no unusual risk for him/her to have cancer? In other words, what is the guarantee that a cancer will not be discovered in this individual, say, after 2 years? To address this question, the confidence on the diagnostic work-up and on the screening test and its principle of operation has to be taken into consideration. If the screening test detects a marker of precancer and cancer with high confidence, then periodic follow-up diagnostic assays may not only be warranted, but also be the appropriate outcome measure with rewarding results. But how does one perform follow-up diagnostic procedures (costing approximately $3825 per cancer patient diagnosed[116]) on individuals that are screen negative? And how long after the initial screen would one compare the values? One cannot simply take an arbitrary period for such a comparison, since it may be too long or too short. If the chosen interval for such a follow-up comparison is too long, it is likely to include some rapidly growing, rather aggressive tumors.[117] In addition, one could also include tumors that developed *de novo,* and therefore at the time of the initial diagnostic procedure was missed. Thus, these cases would not necessarily represent failures on the part of the screening test, and having them included in the comparative study will only underestimate the sensitivity of the test.[117] Likewise, a short interval time is likely to include only rapidly growing tumors and exclude those that are slow growing. Some polyps may never become cancer and those that do may take over 18 years to become cancer,[121] not to forget the fact that the risk of malignancy would also vary depending on the histological grade of the polyp.[122]

The follow-up diagnostic assays should be as complete as possible; for example, the sigmoidoscopy which is commonly used can only visualize the distal left colon, missing over 50% of the lesions that may be in the proximal segments.

V. FINAL COMMENT

The cancer of the colon may arise from the polyps, irrespective of their histological type (although some are more likely than others to harbor malignancy), the flat nonpolypoid mucosa, the divericuli, or any other site wherever the epithelium may be. The risk of cancer becomes higher in those with increased cell proliferation and in various chronic inflammatory diseases of the colon, including foreign body reactions.

The histopathological diagnosis is certainly the most confirmatory for the correct identification of the nature of colonic pathology. However, as I have pointed out earlier, looking for areas that may contain early cancer or precancer may not be easy. There could be situations where the screening assay is positive, but the diagnostic assay is negative due to sampling error. To minimize such false negative results of the diagnostic assay (including that of the histopathological diagnosis) due to improper sampling and the resultant false positivity of the screening assay, we have to devise strategies that would supplement our existing ones, such as identifying areas by special techniques [e.g., Schiller iodine for carcinoma of the uterine cervix or laser-induced fluorescence examination (Chapter 6) preceded by other first-level

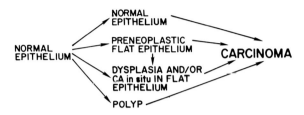

SCHEME 2. Histogenesis of large intestinal carcinoma.

screening assays], and/or identifying individuals that may have the cancer or precancer by following other clues. Exploiting of the expression of various marker substances early during cancer formation gives us such clues and would be one such approach. This naturally leads us to the subject matter of the next chapter.

REFERENCES

1. **Bauer, K. H.,** Mutationstheorie der Geschwulst-Entstehung. Ubergang von Korperzellen, in *Geschwulstzellen durch Genanderung,* Julius Springer, Berlin, 1928.
2. **Berenblum, I.,** Theoretical and practical aspects of the two-stage mechanism of carcinogenesis, The Ernst W. Bertner Memorial Award Lecture, in *Carcinogens, Identification and Mechanisms of Action,* Griffin, A. C. and Shaw, C. R., Raven Press, New York, 1979, 25.
3. **Berenblum, I.,** The modifying influence of dichloro-ethyl sulphide on the induction of tumors in mice by tar, *J. Pathol. Bactriol.,* 32, 425, 1929.
4. **Berenblum, I.,** The mechanism of carcinogenesis: a study of the significance of cocarcinogenic action and related phenomena, *Cancer Res.,* 1, 807, 1941.
5. **Rous, P. and Kidd, J. G.,** Conditional neoplasm and subthreshold neoplastic states, *J. Exp. Med.,* 73, 365, 1941.
6. **Magee, P. N. and Farber, E.,** Toxic liver injury and carcinogenesis. Methylation of rat liver nucleic acid by dimethylnitrosamine *in vivo, Biochem. J.,* 83, 114, 1962.
7. **Narisawa, T., Magadia, N. E., Weisburger, J. H., and Wynder, E. L.,** Promoting effect of bile acids on colon carcinogenesis after intra-rectal instillation of N-methyl-N'-nitro-N-nitrosoguanidine in rats, *J. Natl. Cancer. Inst.,* 53, 1093, 1974.
8. **Pozharisski, K. M.,** The significance of nonspecific injury for colon carcinogenesis in rats, *Cancer Res.,* 35, 3824, 1975.
9. **Barthold, S. W.,** The role of nonspecific injury in colon carcinogenesis, in *Experimental Colon Carcinogenesis,* Autrup, H. and Williams, G. M., Eds., CRC Press, Boca Raton, FL, 1983, 185.
10. **Farber, E. and Cameron, R.,** The sequential analysis of cancer development, *Adv. Cancer Res.,* 31, 125, 1980.
11. **Ames, B. N. and Gold, L. S.,** Too many rodent carcinogens: mitogenesis increases mutagenesis, *Science,* 249, 970, 1990.
12. **Cohen, S. M. and Ellwein, L. B.,** Cell proliferation in carcinogenesis, *Science,* 249, 1007, 1990.
13. **Chakravarthy, A., Elsayed, A., Ullah, A., and Shamsuddin, A. K. M.,** Azoxymethane induced large intestinal carcinogensis in Fischer 344 rats: a two-dimensional dose and time model, *Fed. Proc.,* 46, 744, 1987.
14. **Shamsuddin, A. M.,** Colon organ culture as a model for carcinogenesis, in *Colon Cancer Cells,* Moyer, M. P. and Poste, G. H., Eds., Academic Press, San Diego, CA, 1990, 137.
15. **Moyer, M. P. and Aust, J. B.,** Human colon cells: culture and *in vitro* transformation, *Science,* 224, 1445, 1984.

16. **Moyer, M. P., Dixon, P. S., Culpepper, A. L., and Aust, J. B.,** *In vitro* propagation and characterization of normal, preneoplastic and neoplastic colonic epithelial cells, in *Colon Cancer Cells,* Moyer, M. P. and Poste, G. H., Eds., Academic Press, San Diego, CA, 1990, 85.

17. **Shamsuddin, A. K. M. and Trump, B. F.,** Colon epithelium. III. *In vitro* studies of colon carcinogenesis in Fischer 344 rats. *N*-Methyl-*N*′-nitro-*N*-nitrosoguanidine-induced changes in colon epithelium in explant culture, *J. Natl. Cancer Inst.,* 66, 403, 1981.

18. **Telang, N. T. and Williams, G. M.,** Carcinogen-induced DNA damage and cellular alterations in F344 rat colon organ cultures, *J. Natl. Cancer Inst.,* 68, 1015, 1982.

19. **Weisburger, J. H. and Fiala, E. S.,** Experimental colon carcinogens and their mode of action, in *Experimental Colon Carcinogenesis,* Autrup, H. and Williams, G. M., Eds., CRC Press, Boca Raton, FL, 1983, 27.

20. **Shamsuddin, A. K. M.,** *In vivo* induction of colon cancer: dose and animal species, in *Experimental Colon Carcinogenesis,* Autrup, H. and Williams, G. M., Eds., CRC Press, Boca Raton, FL, 1983, 51.

21. **Wiebecke, B., Lohrs, U., Gimmy, J., and Eder, M.,** Erzeugung von darmtumoren bei mausen durch 1,2-dimethylhydrazin, *Z. Ges.-Exp. Med.,* 149, 277, 1969.

22. **Thurnherr, N., Deschner, E., Stonehill, E., and Lipkins, M.,** Induction of adenocarcinomas of the colon in mice by weekly injections of 1,2-dimethylhydrazine, *Cancer Res.,* 33, 940, 1973.

23. **Deschner, E.,** Experimentally induced cancer of the colon, *Cancer Res.,* 34, 824, 1974.

24. **Maskens, A. P.,** Histogenesis and growth pattern of 1,2-dimethylhydrazine-induced rat colon adenocarcinoma, *Cancer Res.,* 36, 1585, 1976.

25. **Lev, R. and Herp, A.,** Histogenesis of rat colon carcinomas induced by *N*-methyl-*N*-nitrosourea, *J. Natl. Cancer Inst.,* 61, 779, 1978.

26. **Shamsuddin, A. K. M. and Trump, B. F.,** Colon epithelium. II. *In vivo* studies of colon carcinogenesis. Light microscopic, histochemical, and ultrastructural studies of histogenesis of azoxymethane-induced colon carcinomas in Fischer 344 rats, *J. Natl. Cancer Inst.,* 66, 389, 1981.

27. **Pozharisski, K. M.,** Morphology and morphogenesis of experimental epithelial tumors of the intestine, *J. Natl. Cancer Inst.,* 54, 1115, 1975.

28. **Shamsuddin, A. K. M., Sugano, H., and Trump, B. F.,** Morphogenesis of large intestinal carcinoma: its significance in early detection, *GANN Monograph in Cancer Research,* 31, 59, 1986.

29. **Shamsuddin, A. K. M.,** Progression of colon cancer, in *Progressive Stages of Malignant Neoplastic Growth,* Kaiser, H. E., Ed., Martinus Nijhoff, Dordrecht, The Netherlands, Vol. 8, 1989, 64.

30. **Shamsuddin, A. K. M. and Trump, B. F.,** Colon epithelium. I. Light microscopic, histochemical and ultrastructural features of normal colon epithelium of male Fischer 344 rats, *J. Natl. Cancer Inst.,* 66, 375, 1981.

31. **Muto, T., Bussey, H. J. R., and Morson, B. C.,** The evolution of cancer of the colon and rectum, *Cancer,* 36, 2251, 1975.

32. **Shamsuddin, A. M.,** Morphogenesis of colonic carcinoma. Ultrastructural studies of azoxymethane-induced early lesions in colon epithelium of Fischer 344 rats, *Arch. Pathol. Lab. Med.,* 106, 140, 1982.

33. **Shamsuddin, A. K. M., Phelps, P. C., and Trump, B. F.,** Human large intestinal epithelium. Light microscopy, histochemistry and ultrstructure, *Hum. Pathol.,* 13, 790, 1982.

34. **Deschner, E. E.,** Early proliferative defects induced by six weekly injections of 1,3-dimethylhydrazine in epithelial cells of mouse distal colon, *Z. Krebsforsch. Klin. Onkol.,* 91, 205, 1978.

35. **Maskens, A. P.,** Histogenesis of colon glands during postnatal growth, *Arch. Anat.,* 100, 17, 1978.

36. **Maskens, A. P. and Dujardin-Lorts, R.,** Kinetics of tissue proliferation in colorectal mucosa during postnatal growth, *Cell Tissue Kinet.,* 14, 467, 1981.

37. **Autrup, H., Barrett, L. A., Jackson, F. E., Jesudason, M. L., Stoner, G., Phelps, P., and Trump, B. F.,** Explant culture of human colon, *Gastroenterology,* 74, 1248, 1978.

38. **Autrup, H.,** Carcinogenesis studies in human gastrointestinal epithelium, in *Experimental Colon Carcinogenesis,* Autrup, H. and Williams, G. M., Eds., CRC Press, Boca Raton, FL, 1983, 95.

39. **Reiss, B., Telang, N. T., and Williams, G. M.,** The application of organ culture to the study of colon carcinogenesis, in *Experimental Colon Carcinogenesis,* Autrup, H. and Williams, G. M., Eds., CRC Press, Boca Raton, FL, 1983, 83.

40. **Shamsuddin, A. M., Ullah, A., Baten, A., and Hale, E.,** Stability of fecapentaene and its effect on human colon epithelial cells, *Proc. Am. Assoc. Cancer Res.,* 30, 116, 1989.

41. **Shamsuddin, A. M., Ullah, A., Baten, A., and Hale, E.,** Stability of fecapentaene and its carcinogenicity in F-344 rats, *Carcinogenesis,* 12, 601, 1991.

42. **Valerio, M., Fineman, E. L., Bowman, R. L., Harris, C. C., Stoner, G. D., Autrup, H., Trump, B. F., McDowell, E. M., and Jones, R.T.,** Long-term survival of normal human tissues as xenografts in congenitally athymic nude mice, *J. Natl. Cancer Inst.,* 66, 849, 1981.

43. **Sakamoto, K., Resau, J., Shamsuddin, A. M., Yuasa, Y., Hoshino, H., Nakano, G.-I., and Nagamachi, Y.,** Long term explant culture of human colon and a 3-step transformation model for rat colonic epithelium, *Pathobiology,* 1991 (in press).

44. **Danes, B. S. and Sutanto, E.,** Epithelial line from normal human colon mucosa, *J. Natl. Cancer Inst.,* 69, 1271, 1982.
45. **Baten, A., Ullah, A., Resau, J., Trump, B. F., and Shamsuddin, A. M.,** Long-term culture of normal human colon epithelial cells, *Proc. Am. Assoc. Cancer Res.,* 30, 30, 1989.
46. **Rutzky, L. P. and Moyer, M. P.,** Human cell lines in colon cancer research, in *Colon Cancer Cells,* Moyer, M. P. and Poste, G. H., Eds., Academic Press, San Diego, CA, 1990, 155.
47. **Shamsuddin, A. K. M., Weiss, L., Phelps, P. C., and Trump, B. F.,** Colon epithelium. IV. Human colon carcinogenesis. Changes in human colon mucosa adjacent to and remote from carcinomas of the colon, *J. Natl. Cancer Inst.,* 66, 413, 1981.
48. **Shamsuddin, A. M.,** Morphological and Histochemical Studies of the Colonic Epithelium of F-344 Rats Treated with Azoxymethane, Doctoral dissertation, University of Maryland at Baltimore, 1979.
49. **Fenoglio, C. M. and Lane, N.,** The anatomical precursor of colorectal carcinoma, *Cancer,* 34, 819, 1974.
50. **Castleman, B. and Krickstein, H. L.,** Do adenomatous polyps of the colon become malignant?, *N. Engl. J. Med.,* 267, 469, 1962.
51. **Shamsuddin, A. K. M., Bell, H. G., Petrucci, J. V., and Trump, B. F.,** Carcinoma *in situ* and "microinvasive" adenocarcinoma of colon, *Pathol. Res. Pract.,* 167, 374, 1980.
52. **Shamsuddin, A. K. M. and Elias, E. G.,** Rectal mucosa: malignant and premalignant changes after radiation therapy, *Arch. Pathol. Lab. Med.,* 105, 150, 1981.
53. **Shamsuddin, A. K. M.,** Microscopic intraepithelial neoplasia in large bowel mucosa, *Hum. Pathol.,* 13, 510, 1982.
54. **Shamsuddin, A. M., Kato, Y., Kunishima, N., Sugano, H., and Trump, B. F.,** Carcinoma *in situ* in flat mucosa of large intestine; report of a case with significance in strategies for early detection, *Cancer,* 56, 2849, 1985.
55. **Crawford, B. E. and Stromeyer, F. W.,** Small nonpolypoid carcinomas of the large intestine, *Cancer,* 51, 1760, 1983.
56. **Pascal, R.,** Neoplasia in colonic mucosa (letter), *Hum. Pathol.,* 14, 1983.
57. **Shimoda, T., Ikegami, M., Fujisaki, J., Matsui, T., Aizawa, S., and Ishikawa, E.,** Early colorectal carcinoma with special reference to its development *de novo, Cancer,* 64, 1138, 1989.
58. **Lotfi, A. M., Spencer, R. J., Ilstrup, D. M., and Melton, L. J., III,** Colorectal polyps and the risk of subsequent carcinoma, *Mayo Clin. Proc.,* 61, 337, 1986.
59. **Hernandez, F. J. and Fernandez, B. B.,** Mucus-secreting carcinoid tumor in colonic diverticulum. Report of a case, *Dis. Colon Rectum,* 19, 63, 1976.
60. **Camacho, C.,** Amebic granuloma and its relationship to cancer of the cecum, *Dis. Colon Rectum,* 14, 12, 1971.
61. **Barson, A. J. and Kirk, R. S.,** Colonic tuberculosis with carcinoma, *J. Pathol.,* 101, 289, 1970.
62. **Greenstein, A. J., Sacher, D. B., Smith, H., Janowitz, H. D., and Aufses, A. H., Jr.,** Patterns of neoplasia in Crohn's disease and ulcerative colitis, *Cancer,* 46, 403, 1980.
63. **Schilla, F. W.,** Carcinoma in rectal polyp: report of a case in infancy, *Am. J. Surg.,* 88, 659, 1950.
64. **Tun-Hua, L., Min-Chang, C., and Hsien-Chiu, T.,** Malignant change of a juvenile polyp of colon: a case report, *Clin. Med. J.,* 4, 434, 1978.
65. **Lipper, S., Kahn, L. B., and Ackerman, L. V.,** The significance of microscopic invasive cancer in endoscopically removed polyps of the large bowel. A clinicopathological study of 51 cases, *Cancer,* 52, 1691, 1983.
66. **Perzin, K. H. and Bridge, M. F.,** Adenomatous and carcinomatous changes in hamartomatous polyps of the small intestine (Peutz-Jeghers syndrome): report of a case and review of the literature, *Cancer,* 49, 971, 1982.
67. **Morson, B. C. and Dawson, I. P. M.,** *Gastrointestinal Pathology,* Blackwell Scientific Publications, Oxford, U.K., 1979, 648.
68. **Cooper, H. S., Patchefsky, A. S., and Marks, G.,** Adenomatous and carcinomatous changes within hyperplastic colonic epithelium, *Dis. Colon Rectum,* 22, 152, 1979.
69. **Boland, C. R., Montgomery, C. K., and Kim, Y. S.,** Hyperplastic polyps and colorectal cancer, *Lancet,* 1, 480, 1982.
70. **Boland, C. R., Montgomery, C. K., and Kim, Y. S.,** A cancer associated mucin alteration in benign colonic polyps, *Gastroenterology,* 82, 664, 1982.
71. **Skinner, J. M. and Whitehead, R.,** Tumour-associated antigens in polyps and carcinoma of the human large bowel, *Cancer,* 47, 1241, 1981.
72. **Jass, J. R.,** Relation between metaplastic polyp and carcinoma of colon-rectum, *Lancet,* 1, 28, 1983.
73. **Jass, J. R., Filipe, M. I., Abbas, S., Falcon, C. A. G., Wilson, Y., and Lovell, D.,** A morphologic and histochemical study of metaplastic polyps of the colorectum, *Cancer,* 53, 510, 1984.
74. **Foutch, P. G., Mai, H. D., Disario, J. A., Pardy, K., and Hayden, C. T.,** The sentinel hyperplastic polyp — a marker for synchronous neoplasia in the proximal colon, *Am. J. Gastroenterol.,* 85, 1276, 1990.

75. **Urbanski, S. J., Kossakowska, A. E., Marcon, N., and Bruce, W. R.,** Mixed hyperplastic adenomatous polyps — an underdiagnosed entity. Report of a case of adenocarcinoma arising within a mixed hyperplastic adenomatous polyp, *Am. J. Surg. Pathol.,* 8, 551, 1984.

76. **Johnson, D. A., Gurney, M. S., Volpe, R., Jones, D. M., Van Ness, M. M., Chobanian, S. J., Alvarez, J., Buck, J., Kooyman, G., and Cattau, E. L., Jr.,** A prospective study of the prevalence of colonic neoplasms in asymptomatic patients with an age-related risk, *Gastroenterology,* 94, A209, 1988.

77. **Warren S. and Sommers, S. C.,** Pathogenesis of ulcerative colitis, *Am. J. Pathol.,* 25, 657, 1949.

78. **Ekbom, A., Helmick, C., Zack, M., and Adami, H.-O.,** Ulcerative colitis and colon cancer, *N. Engl. J. Med.,* 323, 1228, 1990.

79. **Jones, J. H.,** Colonic cancer and Crohn's disease, *Gut,* 10, 651, 1969.

80. **Weedon, D. D., Shorter, R. G., Ilstrup, D. M., Huizenga, K. A., and Taylor, W. F.,** Crohn's disease and cancer, *N. Engl. J. Med.,* 289, 1099, 1973.

81. **Gyde, S. N., Prior, P., Macartney, J. C., Thompson, H., Waterhouse, J. A. H., and Allen, R. N.,** Malignancy in Crohn's disease, *Gut,* 21, 1024, 1980.

82. **Greenstein, A. J., Sacher, D. B., Smith, H., Janowitz, H. D., and Aufses, A. H.,** A comparison of risk in Crohn's disease and ulcerative colitis, *Cancer,* 48, 2742, 1981.

83. **Ekbom, A., Helmick, C., Zack, M., and Adami, H.-O.,** Increased risk of large-bowel cancer in Crohn's disease with colonic involvement, *Lancet,* 336 (8711), 357, 1990.

84. **Shamsuddin, A. K. M. and Phillips, R. M.,** Preneoplastic and neoplastic changes in colonic mucosa in Crohn's disease, *Arch. Pathol. Lab. Med.,* 105, 283, 1981.

85. **Haggitt, R. C., Appelman, H. D., Correa, P., Fenoglio, C. M., Goldman, H., Hamilton, S. R., Morson, B. C., Ransohoff, D. F., Riddell, R. H., Sommers, S. C., and Yardley, J. H.,** Carcinoma or dysplasia in Crohn's disease (letter), *Arch. Pathol. Lab. Med.,* 106, 308, 1982.

86. **Shamsuddin, A. K. M. and Phillips, R. M.,** Carcinoma or dysplasia in Crohn's disease (in reply), *Arch. Pathol. Lab. Med.,* 106, 308, 1982.

87. **Riddell, R. H., Goldman, H., Ransohoff, D. F., Appelman, H. D., Fenoglio, C. M., Haggitt, R. C., Ahren, C., Correa, P., Hamilton, S. R., Morson, B. C, Sommers, S. C., and Yardley, J. H.,** Dysplasia in inflammatory bowel disease, *Hum. Pathol.,* 14, 931, 1983.

88. **Bacon, H. E., Tse, G. N., and Herabat, T.,** Coexisting carcinoma with peridiverticulitis of the colon, *Dis. Colon Rectum,* 16, 500, 1973.

89. **Winkler, R., Heitman, C., and Otto, H. F.,** Das carcinom am anus praeter-tierexperimentelle unter-suchungen und klinishe beobachtungen, *Langenbecks Arch. Chir.,* 343, 229, 1977.

90. **Sauer, H. D., Winkler, R., Thoma, G., and Mitschke, H.,** Carcinompromotion am anus praeter durch gallensauren — eine tierexperimentelle beobachtungen, *Langenbecks Arch. Chir.,* 350, 255, 1980.

91. **Floyd, C. E., Corley, R. G., and Cohn, I.,** Local recurrence of carcinoma of the colon and rectum, *Am. J. Surg.,* 109, 153, 1965.

92. **Nava, H. R. and Pagana, T. J.,** Postoperative surveillance of colorectal carcinoma, *Cancer,* 49, 1043, 1982.

93. **Tank, E. S., Karsch, D. N., and Lapides, J.,** Adenocarcinoma of the colon associated with ureterosigmoidos-tomy. Report of a case, *Dis. Colon Rectum,* 16, 300, 1973.

94. **Sooriyaarachchi, G. S., Johnson, R. O., and Carbone, P. P.,** Neoplasms of the large bowel following ureterosigmoidostomy, *Arch. Surg.,* 112, 1174, 1977.

95. **Weshler, Z., Sulkes, A., and Rizel, S.,** Carcinoma of the colon following ureterosigmoidostomy, *Dis. Colon Rectum,* 22, 434, 1979.

96. **Crissey, M. M., Steele, G. D., and Gittes, R. F.,** Rat model for carcinogenesis in ureterosigmoidostomy, *Science,* 207, 1079, 1980.

97. **Shindo, K.,** Significance of schistosomiasis japonica in the development of cancer of the large intestine: report of a case and review of the literature, *Dis. Colon Rectum,* 19, 460, 1976.

98. **Ehsanullah, M., Filipe, M. I., and Gazzard, B.,** Mucin secretion in inflammatory bowel disease: correlation with disease activity and dysplasia, *Gut,* 23, 485, 1982.

99. **Ngoi, S. S., Staiano-Coico, L., Godwin, T. A., Wong, R., and DeCosse, J. J.,** Abnormal DNA ploidy and proliferative patterns in superficial colonic epithelium adjacent to colorectal cancer, *Cancer,* 66, 953, 1990.

100. **Bleiberg, H., Buyse, M., and Galand, P.,** Cell kinetic indicators of premalignant stages of colorectal cancer, *Cancer,* 56, 124, 1985.

101. **Deschner, E. E., Lipkin, M., and Solomon, C.,** Study of human rectal epithelial cells *in vitro.* II. ^{3}H-Thymidine incorporation into polyps and adjacent mucosa, *J. Natl. Cancer. Inst.,* 36, 849, 1966.

102. **Preumont, A. M., Stoffels, G. L., and DeReuck, M.,** Nuclear size and nuclear binding of tritiated actino-mycin D into epithelial cells of colon cancer patients with apparently normal colorectal mucosa, *Cancer Res.,* 41, 2529, 1981.

103. **Dawson, P. M., Habib, N. A., Rees, H. C., Williamson, R. C. N., and Wood, C. B.,** Influence of sialomucin at the resection margin on local tumor recurrence and survival of patients with colorectal cancer: a multivariate analysis, *Br. J. Surg.,* 74, 366, 1987.

104. **Fenoglio-Preiser, C. M. and Pascal, R. R.,** Other tumors of the large intestine. I. Epithelial tumors, in *Gastrointestinal and Oesophageal Pathology,* Whitehead, R., Ed., Churchill Livingstone, New York, 1989, 747.

105. **Falterman, K. W., Hill, C. B., Markey, J. C., Fox, J. W., and Cohen, I., Jr.,** Cancer of the rectum and anus — a review of 2313 cases, *Cancer,* 34, 951, 1974.

106. **Symonds, D. A. and Vickery, A. L., Jr.,** Mucinous carcinoma of the colon and rectum, *Cancer,* 37, 1891, 1976.

107. **Pratt, C. B., Rivera, G., Shanks, E., Johnson, W. W., Howarth, C., Terrell, W., and Kumar, P. M.,** Colorectal carcinoma in adolescents. Implications regarding etiology, *Cancer,* 40, 2464, 1977.

108. **Mills, S. E. and Allen, M. S., Jr.,** Colorectal carcinoma in the first three decades of life, *Am. J. Surg. Pathol.,* 3, 443, 1979.

109. **Castro, E. B., Rosen, P. P., and Quan, H. Q.,** Carcinoma of large intestine in patients irradiated for carcinoma of cervix and uterus, *Cancer,* 31, 45, 1973.

110. **Denman, D. L., Kirchner, F. R., and Osborne, J. W.,** Induction of colonic adenocarcinoma in the rat by X-irradiation, *Cancer Res.,* 38, 1899, 1978.

111. **Dukes, C.,** The classification of cancer of the rectum, *J. Pathol. Bacteriol.,* 35, 323, 1932.

112. **Astler, V. B. and Coller, F. A.,** The prognostic significance of direct extension of carcinoma of the colon and rectum, *Ann. Surg.,* 139, 846, 1954.

113. **Wood, D. A., Robbins, G. F., Zippin, C., Lum, D., and Stearns, M.,** Staging of cancer of the colon and cancer of the rectum, *Cancer,* 43, 961, 1979.

114. **Cole, P. and Morrison, A. S.,** Basic issues in population screening for cancer, *J. Natl. Cancer Inst.,* 64, 1263, 1980.

115. **Fink, D. J.,** Facts about colorectal cancer detection, *Ca.,* 33, 366, 1983.

116. **Petrelli, N. J., Palmer, M., Michalek, A., Herrera, L., Mink, I., Bersani, G., and Cummings, K. M.,** Massive screening for colorectal cancer. A single institution's public commitment, *Arch. Surg.,* 125, 1049, 1990.

117. **Frank, J. W.,** Occult-blood screening for colorectal carcinoma: the risks, *Am. J. Prev. Med.,* 1(4), 25, 1985.

118. **Waterhouse, J., Muir, C., Correa, P., and Powell, J.,** *Cancer Incidence in Five Continents,* Vol. 3, I.A.R.C. Sci. Publ. No. 15, International Agency for Research on Cancer, Lyon, 1976.

119. **UICC,** *Cancer Incidence in Five Continents,* Doll, R., Muir, C. S., and Waterhouse, J., Eds., International Union Against Cancer, Springer Verlag, Berlin, 1970.

120. **Frank, J. W.,** Occult-blood screening for colorectal carcinoma: the yield and the cost, *Am. J. Prev. Med.,* 1(5), 18, 1985.

121. **Kozuka, S., Nogake, M., Ozeki, T., Ozeki, T., and Masumori, S.,** Premalignancy of the mucosal polyp in the large intestine. II. Estimation of the periods required for malignant transformation of mucosal polyps, *Dis. Colon Rect.,* 18, 494, 1975.

122. **Kozuka, S.,** Premalignancy of the mucosal polyp in the large intestine. I. Histologic gradation of the polyp on the basis of epithelial pseudostratification and glandular branching, *Dis. Colon Rect.,* 18, 483, 1975.

Chapter 3

MARKERS OF PRECANCER AND CANCER

I. INTRODUCTION

A. MARKER

Markers are physical and/or behavioral characteristics that are invaluable in the identification of living organisms as well as nonliving substances or processes. Like most other cancers, the physical appearance and biologic behavior of cancers of the large intestine are usually obvious, making it easy (albeit, painful) for most in the health profession as well as the patient to recognize the existence of the disease. Thus, we need markers that are expressed or detected beforehand to help identify the disease early. The markers that may be expressed during the early stages of cancer of the large intestine may also be physical and behavioral or functional. Because of the overlapping nature of the modern technologies and divergence of properties, any attempt to classify them in a rigid system can hardly be perfect. In any event, for easy understanding, one may look at the markers of precancer and cancer as:

A.   Structural (pathologic morphology)
     1.   Endoscopic
     2.   Microscopic (light & electron)
B.   Functional (pathobiology and molecular pathology)
     1.   Altered gene expression (carbohydrates and *onc* gene products)
     2.   Altered enzyme and metabolite
     3.   Altered cell proliferation
     4.   Altered immunogenicity

It is obvious even from the above, somewhat overly simplistic classification, that there are several overlaps. For example, the altered immunogenicity is due to altered structure and it either reflects or brings about altered function. Thus, structure and function are fundamentally integrated to one another and are indivisible. Any attempt to further dissect and classify is therefore fraught only with overlap and perhaps confuses the issue. I shall therefore describe the markers under the headings that best describe their importance and relevance.

Since the description of the various markers entails a basic knowledge of the pathology of the large intestine as it relates to the genesis of precancer and cancer, for the benefit of those readers who are less familiar with the subject, I shall briefly touch upon the subject.

B. PATHOLOGY OF THE PRECANCER AND CANCER

Much of the pathology of the precancer and cancer has been discussed in Chapter 2. To summarize, the cancers of the large intestine are predominantly epithelial, hence called carcinomas. Since the normal epithelium lining the intestine is glandular in nature, the vast majority of carcinomas are adenocarcinomas. The anal canal is lined by squamous epithelium and thus squamous cell carcinomas are commonly seen in that area. Cancers arising from specialized cells that are situated within the layer of lining epithelium, such as the endocrine cells, give rise to carcinoid tumors.

The precancers of the large intestine can be arbitrarily looked as (1) precancerous lesions which are strict morphological entities and (2) various clinical entities that predispose to cancer, hence precancerous conditions.

1. Precancerous Lesions

The most notable of these are the polyps which are masses of tissue that project into the lumen of the intestine; however, not all projecting masses or polyps carry a high risk of advancing to cancer. The common hyperplastic polyps, seen in ~75% of people over the age of 40 years, are rarely associated with morphological evidence of malignancy. Thus, they are not considered to be precancerous although they share many biochemical markers with the cancer. This issue will be discussed further in a subsequent section (Section II.B). The readers are cautioned that in the absence of scientific evidence showing transformation of these various lesions to cancer, the present day dogma has been adapted from mere histopathological observation of the association between the two; that is, cancerous foci in the polyps. As any student of biology would predict, the chances of observing such association will depend heavily on the extent of sampling (e.g., how many 5-μm sections were examined from a 1-cm diameter polyp?), besides the training, bias, and the motivation of the investigator.

In any event, the polyps that are considered to be associated with a high risk of malignancy are called neoplastic polyps, which include the tubular adenomas and the villous adenomas. The former is quite common with a lesser degree of association with cancer, while the latter is rare but is quite frequently associated with histopathologic foci of malignancy. A considerable overlap of histopathological features is beginning to be appreciated between the hyperplastic polyps, tubular adenomas, and villous adenomas;[1] a fact that supports my contention that as we examine these lesions more and more carefully, the dogma will have to be revised (Chapter 2). Aside from the easily recognizable polyps, microscopic foci of carcinomas and dysplasias are observed in the flat nonpolypoid epithelium of the large intestine and these have been well documented in the literature[2-5] (please refer to Chapter 2 for details). The harsh reality is the difficulty to recognize and detect these lesions early on, before the process spreads further.

2. Precancerous Conditions

The dogma in carcinogenesis says that the formation of cancer is a multistep process whereby the normal cells are "initiated" by carcinogenic agents and, subsequently, various factors "promote" the initiated cells to neoplastic cells and then cause "progression". A fundamental process in cancer formation is that the normal cells, as they become cancer, undergo uncontrolled cell division, accounting for the mass of tumor tissue. Inasmuch as cell division is vital for the very process of cancer formation, conditions that favor cell division would logically favor neoplastic growth; a sundry of chemicals that are released or genes that are activated during these conditions, may additionally enhance the neoplastic process in the large intestine.[6] Diverse chronic disease processes that continuously stimulate cell proliferation therefore carry with them a high risk of malignant transformation. Most commonly, these are ulcerative colitis and Crohn's disease (also called regional enteritis). However, as explained above, other so-called nonspecific injuries (colostomy, ureterosigmoidostomy, suture granuloma, diverticulosis, etc.) would also enhance the risk of malignant transformation in the colon.

II. CONVENTIONAL MORPHOLOGICAL MARKERS

This term refers to the morphological tools and techniques that have been conventionally used, such as the light microscopic, electron microscopic (both transmission and scanning), or endoscopic visualization. This is to separate other more modern techniques where the microscopy is more advanced (such as scanning tunneling microscopy) or where it is combined with immunology, hybridization (e.g., *in situ* hybridization), etc.

A. MICROSCOPIC

1. Abnormal Crypts

Using a conventional light microscope and the popular hematoxylin and eosin (H & E) stain, I had first reported the presence of various subtle abnormalities in the mucosa of human large intestine that harbors cancers. These are: dilatation of the colonic crypts, distortion, branching or hyperdistention of the crypts, hypercellularity, atypia, and "dysplastic" changes in the crypts.[7] Lately these changes have also been observed in humans by others;[8] but they had been and still are, considered by some as "nonspecific" changes.[8] First, these abnormalities are not present in the normal control individuals.[9] Secondly, even a cursory comparison with the morphology of the rodent colon undergoing carcinogenesis demonstrates the striking similarity of these lesions with the precancerous changes between the human lesion and their counterpart in the experimental models.[10-13] Furthermore, these same lesions are seen quite commonly in the diseases and conditions that are known to be associated with a high risk of cancer of the large intestine, such as ulcerative colitis, Crohn's disease, neoplastic polyps, etc.[14,15]

Aside from the above data obtained in my laboratory, further evidence of the pre-neoplastic nature of these abnormal crypts come from the more recent studies of McLellan and Bird,[16,17] Roncucci et al.[18] and Pretlow et al.[19] McLellan and Bird have demonstrated in the murine model that the aberrant crypts are induced in a dose-dependent manner only by the carcinogens; none of the noncarcinogenic substances tested had induced the abnormal or "aberrant" crypts.[16,17] Using the technique of methylene blue staining as introduced by Bird and co-workers,[16,17] Roncucci et al.[18] demonstrate a similar presence of abnormal, often dysplastic crypt in mucosa remote from other neoplasms in the human colon, altogether lending support to the field-effect theory (*vide infra*).

However, one must not assume that all these precancerous or pre-neoplastic changes will invariably progress to malignancy; some of them do and others do not. The same is true for the neoplastic polyps which are unquestionably precancerous lesions; but only a small proportion of them are associated with malignancy. The fact that malignancy is not seen in 100% of the neoplastic polyps makes the statement that not all precancerous lesions will progress to cancer. Whether or not precancerous changes or lesions will progress to malignancy will depend on a variety of factors.

2. Micronuclei Markers

Another marker that has been noted by light microscopy is the so-called micronuclei. McLellan and Bird,[16,17] and Heddle et al.,[20] and Wargovich et al.[21] described the presence of small nuclear fragments in the colonic epithelial cells of animals treated with either chemical or physical carcinogens. Both these markers (viz. the abnormal crypts and micronuclei) are interesting for a variety of reasons; however, the translation of these markers to practical screening tests is another matter. First, in both situations, a biopsy of the large intestinal epithelium must be taken, which will have to be processed for microscopic examination and then evaluated by professionals trained and experienced in this matter. Aside from the invasive nature of the sampling, the time delay and the cost would be prohibitory.

3. Ultrastructure Markers

With the introduction of electron microscopy, as with any other new tool or technology, investigators started to look for markers that would characterize and hence discriminate between cancer and normal. A fairly extensive body of literature exists as regards the detailed transmission and scanning electron microscopic morphology of cancer and polyps.[22] Since, a morphological distinction between these various lesions are usually obvious by light microscopy, the ultrastructural morphology of the cancer and polyp as markers has been noncontributory for early diagnosis. Dawson et al.[23] and Dawson and Filipe[24] have reported that the mucosal cells in between the polyps of patients with familial polyposis syndrome are characterized by dense, apical vesicles in the mucous cells as opposed to the normal from the rectum. This was exciting at the beginning because of the potential usefulness in identifying high-risk individuals by rectal biopsy, the very tedious and time-consuming process of electron microscopic preparation notwithstanding. Subsequent studies in our laboratories have dampened the hope by demonstrating that the reported ultrastructural features are normal characteristics of the human ascending and transverse colon, but not of the rectum.[9]

There have also been studies of the scanning electron microscopic morphology of the cancer and polyps,[25,26] One could likewise argue that the time and cost of scanning electron microscopy could not be justified for diagnostic screening of any population, high-risk or otherwise. However, consider this: the relatively low magnification at which the scanning electron microscope visualizes the surface topography may train our eyes for recognition of subtle abnormalities by endoscopy or endoscopy coupled with microscopy (such as the colpomicroscope used in the early detection of the precancer and cancer of the uterine cervix).

This takes us naturally to the next group of markers, the endoscopic markers.

B. ENDOSCOPIC MARKERS

Endoscopic recognition of the cancer or polyp may be fairly straightforward, but the accuracy depends on the training, skill, etc. besides the mood of the operator since it is subjective recognition of a lesion. The problem arises with small polyps and microscopic carcinomas. The advocacy for, and the actual usage of, endoscopy in screening for large intestinal cancer and precancer is discussed in the next chapter. My co-workers and I had described a case of *in situ* carcinoma in the flat nonpolypoid mucosa of the colon in a young Japanese which was detected by colonoscopy.[5] Thus, it is not inconceivable that subtle lesions could be recognized by endoscopy, of course, the final diagnosis of any such suspicious lesion must be confirmed by histopathologic examination.

C. MISCELLANEOUS MARKERS

The so-called hyperplastic polyps are also known as metaplastic polyps. Despite occasional reports of carcinoma arising from them, most consider them to have very little or no malignant potential. Recently, there has been a resurgence of interest surrounding the hyperplastic polyp and not without justification. There are several markers that are commonly shared by both hyperplastic polyps and cancers.[27] It is intriguing that in spite of expressing several functional characteristics of malignancy, they progress to cancer presumably only on rare occasion. It would be worthwhile to study the factor(s), if any that prevent them from progressing to cancer. Ansher et al.[28] and Foutch et al.[29] reported that the presence of hyperplastic polyp is an indication of the synchronous existence of the neoplastic polyps in the proximal segments of the large intestine, which carry a higher risk of malignancy. Compared to a 15% prevalence rate for a neoplastic polyp, 49% of patients harboring hyperplastic polyps also had synchronous neoplastic polyps.[28]

III. CYTOSKELETAL MARKERS

The cytoskeleton is the anastomosing system of intracellular structural framework, composed of microfilaments, intermediate filaments, microtubules and various binding proteins, enzymes, etc. Similar to the skeletal system in the human body, these components are responsible for cellular movement either as a whole or in part (e.g., phagocytosis, secretion, or intracellular transport as in the neuronal axons), cell shape, force production and transduction, cell division, etc.

During cellular transformation, there is alteration in organization of the cytoskeleton and altered expression of cytoskeletal protein.[30] The microvilli of the apical plasma membrane of intestinal cells are supported by the actin microfilaments of the cytoskeleton. Villin, a 95,000 M_r protein binds to actin in a calcium-dependent process and is found in the epithelial cells of the intestine and proximal tubules of kidney, and is absent in tumors arising from cells in which it is normally absent. Using an enzyme-linked immunosorbent assay, Dudouet et al.[31] tested the sera of 788 patients and controls and report a 50.5% sensitivity for colorectal cancers. The overall specificity for malignant neoplasms of the digestive tract was 94.5%. Thus, villin as a marker has good potential in diagnosis and monitoring of individuals with colorectal and other gastrointestinal tract malignancies.

IV. GLYCOCONJUGATES

The three basic structural and functional units of the living cells (carbohydrates, lipids, and proteins) are intimately related; quite often, carbohydrate moiety is covalently linked (conjugated) with either the lipid (glycolipid) or the protein (glycoprotein). Carbohydrates are composed of carbon (*carbo-*), hydrogen, and oxygen (*-hydrate*). The simplest carbohydrates are *monosaccharides* or simple sugars with the following generic composition: $(CH_2O)_n$ and n = 4, 5, 6, or 7. Carbohydrates in the DNA and RNA are pentoses since they have five carbon atoms; those that have six carbon atoms are hexoses (e.g., glucose, galactose, mannose, fucose, and fructose). These are the most important constituents of the glycoconjugates. While monosaccharides are single carbohydrate units, *disaccharides* are two monosaccharides joined together by glycosidic bonds (the common cane sugar is sucrose, which is glucose plus fructose). *Oligosaccharides* contain up to ten monosaccharide units and *polysaccharides* contain many monosaccharide units that may be in long, linear or more commonly branched chains, again linked by glycosidic bonds between the two adjacent sugars. There can be many different types of glycosidic bonds between two monosaccharides and the standard expression (you will commonly find in the literature) is as follows: $\alpha(1\rightarrow1)$, $\alpha(1\rightarrow4)$, $\beta(1\rightarrow3)$, $\beta(1\rightarrow6)$, etc. for galactose and glucose, where α or β indicates the conformation at the 1 carbon in

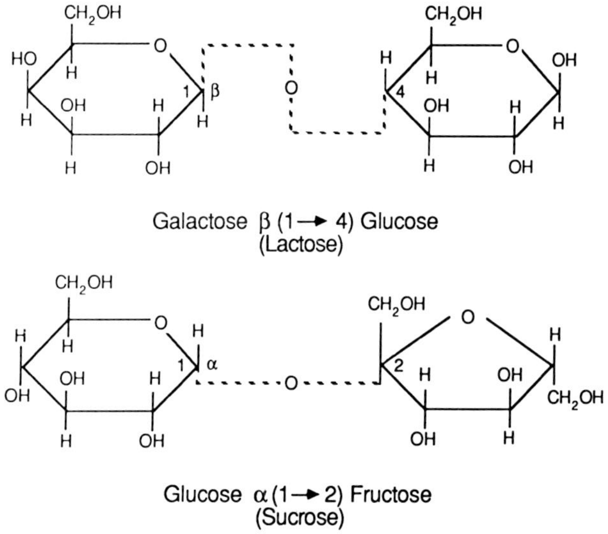

Galactose β (1→ 4) Glucose
(Lactose)

Glucose α (1→ 2) Fructose
(Sucrose)

SCHEME 1.

galactose, the arrow to the second number indicates to which carbon position in glucose it is bound. The scheme below illustrates the different types of linkages between carbohydrates.

The glycoconjugates are rather important and ubiquitous in the cell and extracellular spaces. They are an important constituent of the cell membrane, vital to signal recognition, transduction, cell to cell contact, differentiation, adhesion, immunological processing (antibodies are glycoprotein molecules), etc. They are also abundant in the various secretions in the body, commonly called mucus.

A. MUCIN HISTOCHEMICAL MARKERS

Mucus, the slimy secretion of the gastrointestinal tract is principally composed of water and mucopolysaccharide (mucin). The latter is a glycoprotein, the carbohydrate residues being covalently bound to the central protein core. Not only are the glycoproteins present in the gastrointestinal tract mucus, but they are also present in cell membranes (*vide infra*) and serum (antibodies). The carbohydrate side chains are of relatively short length (oligosaccharide) and show marked variation in the number of sugar residues and complexity of branching; the outer-most (or terminal) sugar in the chain is often the negatively charged *N*-acetylneuraminic acid (or sialic acid), resulting in a net negative charge on the surface of the glycoprotein. The sialic acid in the gastrointestinal mucus is usually linked to the subterminal galactose and, on occasion, to internal *N*-acetylgalactosamine (GalNAc). The sugar residues of the glycoprotein may be bound to the protein by either *O*-link (bound to hydroxyl oxygen of serine and threonine) or by *N*-link (bound to amide nitrogen of asparagine).

In contrast to the soluble proteins of the cytosol which are not glycosylated, the glycoproteins are destined for secretion or transportation to other cell sites such as the plasma membrane, Golgi, lysosome, etc. The glycosylation appears to take place in the luminal side of the endoplasmic reticulum where the oligosaccharide chains are added to the growing polypeptide chain.

In pathology laboratories, the center of most biomedical research until recent years, many of the early discoveries were accomplished mostly by histopathological, histochemical, and less often, biochemical techniques. Perhaps because "seeing is believing", the simplicity of the techniques, and the fondness of pathologists for the microscope, histochemical techniques done on tissue sections yielding colorful results had been popular, notwithstanding the fact that the principles of many of the classical histochemical techniques are ill understood. Besides, the tissue preparation does not often undergo the rigorous quality control used in most biochemical experiments. The length of time elapsed between removal of tissue from the body to fixation (to halt autolytic changes), the type of fixative used, the process of dehydration, infiltration by paraffin, instability of many of the compounds, etc. may result in alteration of the biochemical structure of the marker substances in question, with erroneous results. Be that as it may, the classical histochemical techniques nevertheless have yielded some important clues to our understanding of the emergence of markers, particularly the mucin markers. By using the periodic acid-Schiff (PAS) sequence, the mucin has traditionally been classified into either neutral or acidic, the neutral being PAS reactive (magenta to red colored product). The acidic mucopolysaccharides are commonly identified by their reactivity with basic dyes such as alcian blue. Using alcian blue-PAS sequence, one could first stain all the acidic mucin and then visualize the remaining neutral mucin if any. Examination of the normal human large intestine by this sequence produced some surprises; the mucus in the crypts of ascending colon show a mixture of acidic and neutral mucin with a predominance of the latter, while that of the rectum is almost exclusively acidic in nature[9] (Plate 1, see color plates*). The acidic mucin can, in turn, be differentiated into sulfomucin and sialomucin, and the latter can be further subclassified into *N*- or *O*-acetyl groups.[32] The carbohydrate residues of the mucous glycoprotein often contain terminal sialic acid molecules which may be quantitatively altered in malignancy. Quantitative analyses of sialic acid show an increased amount in primary and

* See color plates following page 102.

metastatic cancers as compared to normal.[33] While histochemical demonstration of sialic acid in tissue sections by modifications of PAS techniques such as PB/KOH/PAS or PT/KOH/PAS[34,35] demonstrate a reduction or loss of *O*-acetylated sialic acids in patients at high risk of colon cancer,[36,37] more accurate biochemical analysis shows a highly variable and only a slightly lower level in colonic adenocarcinomas than normal adult colon.[38] It is also possible that sialic acids may undergo rearrangement in terms of their location on the other sugar residues within the carbohydrate backbone in malignancy. Whatever the case may be, the exact role of the sialic acid molecule and its structural and/or positional alterations during carcinogenesis remains enigmatic.[39]

In addition to classical histochemical staining, newer approaches such as lectin binding and immunohistochemical procedures have been developed that can yield more specific information regarding the composition of the sugars in the mucin *(vide infra)*.

Filipe and co-workers first noted differences in histochemical nature of colonic mucin between carcinomas and the normal appearing epithelium in humans[40] and in animals experimentally induced to bear colon carcinomas.[41] The reason for and the exact significance of the presence of such altered cancer-type mucin in "normal"-appearing epithelium was not known at that time, particularly in light of the dogma that all colon cancers arise from polyps only. Studies in my laboratory on the histogenesis of carcinomas however offered the field effect hypothesis[7] and it is now possible to rationalize these observed changes in light of the experimental data. In short, there are specific biochemical alterations in the mucous glycoconjugate during cancer formation. These changes are seen both in human precancer and cancer, and in experimental models *in vivo* and *in vitro* (Plate 2, see color plates*).

Note that the mucus in both the rat and human colon is sulfomucin that appears brown black with high iron diamine-alcian blue (HID-AB) stain (above left and opposite left), whereas early after carcinogenic stimuli, either *in vivo*[10] (above right) or *in vitro*[11] (opposite above) there is a shift in the nature of mucus — from normal brown black sulfomucin to abnormal blue colored sialomucin. Identical to the experimental models, human colon mucosa either adjacent to cancer or even as far remote as the distal margin of resection shows areas of abnormal sialomucin, with or without abnormal morphology of the crypts[7] (opposite right). This comparison of the data between experimental models and human disease and a bit of extrapolation (done as shown in the schematic diagram of Chapter 2) led to the synthesis of the hypothesis that mucin alteration is perhaps one of the earliest phenotypic expression of genomic damage to the colonic epithelial cells, even before conventional histopathological changes of cancer or precancer can be recognized.[7]

The presence of sialomucin has however been demonstrated in a wide of variety of human and rodent neoplasias, including melanoma, mammary adenocarcinoma, hepatoma, and gall bladder carcinomas,[42-45] thus, sialomucin may not be organ specific, but its presence only in cancer and precancer (except in normal stomach) has earned its place as a cancer marker. It may be worthwhile repeating the precautionary remark that because of the differences in sensitivity, molecular preservation and other unknown factors, between biochemical and histochemical determinations, the term sialomucin is a loose one at best and extreme caution must be exercised in assuming that the sialomucin as detected histochemically is the same as that analyzed biochemically. Simply put, I am not sure we fully understand the exact composition of "sialomucin", much less its function.

B. GLYCOPROTEINS AND GLYCOLIPIDS

As opposed to the rather "crude" sulfomucin and sialomucin, the glycoproteins and glycolipids are rather well-characterized molecules. As mentioned before, the sugar residues may be *O*-Linked, which are generally shorter than the *N*-linked ones, the former usually containing one to three sugar residues. Glycolipids have a variable number of sugars that are linked to the hydroxyl group of the lipid sphingosine, the sugar *N*-acetylneuraminic acid (sialic

---

* See color plates following page 102.

acid) being common. Glycolipids are most commonly found inserted in the lipid bilayer of the cell membrane, with the polar carbohydrate chains facing the exterior. The carbohydrate side chains of the glycolipids and glycoproteins facing the exterior of the cell serve as the antenna for the cell, except that they are responsible for lot more of the cellular functions than your garden variety television antenna or even the "cable". Given the fact that the composition of the carbohydrates remain the same, alteration in their branching pattern merely say $\beta(1\rightarrow3)$ to $(1\rightarrow4)$ could confer a different antigenicity. Thus, other less subtle alterations (in branching pattern, composition, sequence of carbohydrates, etc.) conceivably result in major changes in antigenicity and, along with that, the function of the molecule which in turn alters the behavior of the cell as a whole. Thanks to the ever increasing power of monoclonal antibody and newer domain antibody techniques, it is now possible to dissect these minor alterations in chemical composition.

1. Blood Group Antigen-Related Glycoconjugates

The glycoproteins and glycolipids constitute the blood group antigens, the composition of the crucial carbohydrate moieties being genetically determined. The research and the resultant literature on carbohydrate markers extensively refers to blood group substances. Thus follows a simple introduction to them. The A, B, and O antigens of ABO blood groups are structurally related oligosaccharides bound to lipids or proteins (i.e., glycolipids and glycoproteins).

O antigen: Gal-GlcNAc-Gal-Glc — lipid/protein
               |
               Fuc

A antigen: GalNAc-Gal-GlcNAc-Gal-Glc — lipid/protein
                   |
                 Fuc

B antigen: Gal-Gal-GlcNAc-Gal-Glc — lipid/protein
               |
               Fuc

Gal = galactose, GalNAc = *N*-acetylgalactosamine, Fuc = fucose, Glc = glucose, GlcNAc = *N*-acetylglucosamine

Note that the three blood group antigens are structurally related, the A and B antigens differ from the O antigen by having an extra GalNAc (A) or a Gal residue (B). The immune system in the body can recognize these subtle alterations in the chemical structures and produce antibodies specific for each of them. Inasmuch as subtle alteration often results in incompatible life-threatening immune reaction, the science of it has helped us in dissecting these very obscure changes taking place during carcinogenesis, thus enabling us to identify markers for the preservation of life. Note that the Le^b and Le^y are simple positional isomers, the bold numbers indicating the changes in position of linkage.

Le^b: Gal——$\beta(1\rightarrow3)$——GlcNAc—R
         | |
        Fuc $\alpha1\rightarrow2$ Fuc $\alpha1\rightarrow4$

Le^y: Gal——$\beta(1\rightarrow\mathbf{4})$——GlcNAc—R
         | |
        Fuc $\alpha1\rightarrow2$ Fuc $\alpha1\rightarrow\mathbf{3}$

We now know that the epithelial cells of the human large intestine also express the antigenic determinants of the major blood groups, with variation during the embryonic development, birth, and cancer formation. In addition to the altered and perhaps inappropriate expression of these blood group determinants (or antigens), there is also expression of new carbohydrate markers during cancer formation.[46]

Immunocytochemical studies, mostly from Young Kim's laboratory, have revealed that the proximal and distal colon in the fetus share the same antigenicity as that of A, B, H, Le^a, Le^b, and Le^x blood groups. Following birth, A, B, H, Le^b, and Le^x disappear (A, B, H, and Le^b persist in the proximal colon), only to reappear in polyps (adenomatous and hyperplastic) and cancers.[47-50] Note the expression of these markers in hyperplastic polyps which are considered non-neoplastic in nature. This similarity of the carbohydrate markers expressed in malignant and premalignant tissues in colon to the antigenic determinants of blood group substances on the red blood cell has caused many an investigator to call these markers "blood group antigens" or similar terms. This may be somewhat confusing, if not misleading. I shall therefore try to refrain from using that term henceforth and I recommend my readers to do the same.

Sialosyl Le^a, which is simply a sialic acid linked to the terminal galactose of Le^a, is present in the normal fetal small and large intestine but not in the normal adult colon,[51,52] and is expressed to a variable degree in adenomatous polyps and cancers of the large intestine. Because of its detection by the monoclonal antibody CA 19-9, Sialosyl Le^a is often referred as such.[53] Elevated levels of Sialosyl Le^a in the serum are also found in patients with large intestinal cancer.[54,55] Kim et al.[56] have also demonstrated immunogenicity to Le^y and extended Le^y-related antigens to be oncofetal markers in the colon.

When a sialic acid is attached to the terminal galactose of the disaccharide Gal-β(1→3)-GalNAc, its antigenicity is similar to that of the MN blood group. Treatment of normal red blood cells with neuraminidase to remove the sialic acid results in its unmasking. The disaccharide Gal-β(1→3)-GalNAc alone (also called T antigen, Tag, or Thomsen-Friedenreich antigen) is not expressed in the normal colon, but seen in cancer.[57-62] Carbohydrate residues related to Gal-β(1→3)-GalNAc, Tn and sialosyl Tn also appear to be oncofetal markers.[63] While most of the studies on Gal-β(1→3)-GalNAc were done in human tissues (cancer, precancer, and normal control), that done in my laboratory has demonstrated that it is also expressed in experimental models during carcinogenesis, in precancerous lesions in human, and in the normal-appearing mucosa remote from cancer of the colon in conformity with the field effect theory (*vide infra*).[59,60] I have exploited these features, resulting in the development of screening tests that are described in Chapters 5 and 6.

Is Gal-β(1→3)-GalNAc as a marker restricted to colon cancers? No, it appears to be a marker expressed during cancer formation in various tissues and not just the large intestine.[64–69] Springer[65] estimates that approximately 90% of human carcinomas express Gal-β(1→3)-GalNAc.

2. Carcinoembryonic Antigen (CEA)

By far, the CEA has been the most widely known glycoconjugate marker; it was first isolated from carcinoma of the colon in 1965 by Gold and Freedman.[70] It was so named because of its presence both in carcinoma and fetal tissue. It was at first thought to be a colon cancer specific marker, but similar to the Gal-β(1→3)-GalNAc, its expression has been demonstrated in a variety of other cancerous; and unlike Gal-β(1→3)-GalNAc (so far), in normal tissues as well.[71,72]

Exploitation of CEA expression in cancer has resulted in development of assays for its identification in the serum (see Chapter 4). Fecal CEA determinations have also been recently advocated.[73] One of the major problems with CEA as a marker is not its presence in other tumors, but in non-tumorous conditions and even in normal. Another major problem is its immunologic similarity with many other glycoproteins, resulting in cross-reactivity.[74] However, the quest for finding better antibodies has not stopped and we shall have wait to see the result of some of the newer antibodies.[75] At the moment, CEA is not used as a marker of precancer and cancer, but rather to monitor patients following resection of colon cancer for metachronous and/or metastatic cancer.[76,77]

3. Miscellaneous Components of Mucus

A host of antigenic determinants of the mucous glycoconjugates (mostly glycoproteins) have been immunologically identified in the cancer tissue and/or serum of patients with colorectal cancer and are commonly referred to by their abbreviated names. CMA (Colonic Mucoprotein Antigen) is a 1.5×10^7-Da antigen that has been demonstrated to be present both in the goblet cell mucus and in the secreted mucus. CMA is expressed in 60% of colon carcinomas and rarely in noncolonic carcinomas; however, its expression appears to be limited to well-differentiated carcinomas only, since poorly differentiated ones rarely show immunoreactivity with the antibody.[78,79]

Colon Specific Antigen (CSAp) was first identified by Pant et al.[80,81] with the use of a goat polyclonal antiserum following absorption with nongastrointestinal tissues. Similar to the CMA, approximately 60% of patients with advanced colorectal cancer have elevated serum CSAp titers. Gold et al.[82] recently reported the isolation of a murine monoclonal antibody Mu-9 which appears to be more specific than the previous ones, the rate of positive reaction with colonic tumors however remains the same as that of serum (i.e., 60%).

Colon-Associated Antigen (CAA) is a 200-kDa antigen isolated from the colonic cell membrane and has been reported to be expressed in approximately 90% of carcinomas.[83] A mucin antigen identified by the antibody G9 has been shown to react immunocytochemically with 70% of colonic carcinomas, albeit only 1 of 6 poorly differentiated cancers showed immunoreactivity.[84] The antibody appears to be organ specific since breast, lung, and ovarian tumors do not elicit a positive reaction.[84]

Bara et al. have worked extensively on mucin (M) antigens[85-87] which consist of three apparently different components M_{1-3}. M_1 is expressed in the distal large intestine, early during experimental colon carcinogenesis and is found in approximately 55% of proximal colon cancers; however, only 12% of cancers in the distal colon express this antigen. The experimental data and that of expression of M_1 antigen in 66% of distal colon polyps indicate that in the distal large intestine, the marker appears early during neoplastic transformation and is suppressed during later stages of progression to malignancy.[88]

Other mucin-related antigenic markers include MAM-6,[89] and TAG-72, identified by the monoclonal antibody named B72.3.[90-92] The usefulness of these have to be determined in the coming years.[92]

C. IDENTIFICATION OF CARBOHYDRATE MARKERS

The carbohydrate markers may be detected in the colorectal tissue or in the blood. A common line of thought is that if the marker is expressed in the cancer tissues, it is likely to be detected in the blood, notwithstanding the fact that by the time a cancer marker has reached blood from the colon, the cancer itself is also perhaps not restricted to the confines of the colonic mucosa either. Thus, while emergence of a marker in the blood may serve as a diagnostic clue, it is may also serve as an indicator of not so good a prognosis.

Testing of blood for markers has been popular both to the physicians and to the patients; the latter often is impressed that some important test has been done. Thus, the all-time popular blood tests have been well standardized over the years. What is not standardized are the detection of the markers in tissue sections. The literature is full of reports with conflicting claims regarding the presence of markers, often resulting in severe frustration on the part of

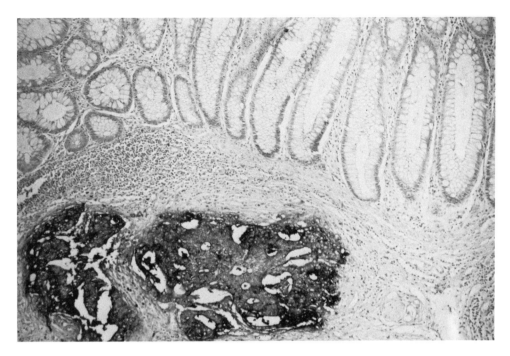

FIGURE 1. Immunoperoxidase study of an adenocarcinoma of the colon reacted with anti-CEA antibody. Note that the infiltrating malignant glandular components show intense reactivity, while the overlying noncarcinomatous tissue is nonreactive.

the investigators. Kathryn McKenzie, a medical student at the University of Glasgow, Scotland, came to my laboratory in the summer of 1986 to do a project on the carbohydrate and oncogene markers of precancer and cancer of the colon. While many a investigator has abandoned CEA to be a nonspecific tissue marker, Kathryn found that (besides other interesting observations) appropriate fixation of tissue is crucial in investigating the expression of CEA in the tissues. When fixed in the Universal Fixative (a mixture of 4% formaldehyde and 1% glutaraldehyde),[93] immunoreactivity to CEA cannot be demonstrated in the normal human colon epithelial mucin. On the other hand, a rather intense immunoreactivity can be seen in cancer (Figure 1) and polyps[60] (Figure 2). This differential expression demonstrated by using a specific fixative indicates the importance of tissue preservation in interpretation of the results, particularly in immunocytochemistry. It is quite possible that the antigenic determinants are variably suppressed by different fixatives and conditions of tissue processing.

I cannot help but remind you one more time of the importance of the appropriate control, the most important of all, the normal human colon. One must be extremely careful as to the source of the normal.[9] Now let us consider the techniques.

1. Immunocytochemistry

Immunological detection of antigenic tissue markers has been popular because it allows indirect visualization of the markers on the tissues. Simply put, a specific antibody against the marker (primary antibody) is added; a second antibody (against the primary antibody) conjugated with an enzyme, dye, or heavy metal is then reacted with the primary antibody. The fluorescence, enzyme, or the heavy metal (e.g., gold for immunoelectron microscopy) allows indirect visualization of the antigen. Two common techniques are immunofluorescence and immunoperoxidase, the former uses fluorescent dye conjugated to a second antibody to the primary anti-marker antibody. In immunoperoxidase, an enzyme (usually horseradish peroxi-

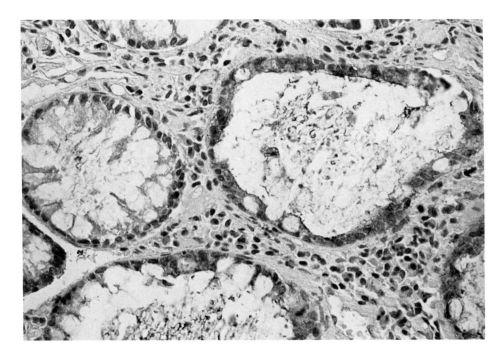

FIGURE 2. A dilated crypt (upper right) in an adenomatous polyp showing moderate immunoreactivity with anti-CEA antibody. (From McKenzie, K. J., Purnell, D. M., and Shamsuddin, A. M., *Hum. Pathol.*, 18, 1282, 1987. With permission.)

dase) is used instead of the fluorescent dye. Each of these has its own advantages and limitations, the peroxidase technique being simpler, can be done on archival tissues and do not require fluorescent microscopy, and therefore the most popular. I am afraid that in the process the assay may have been rendered less accurate, as exemplified by Kathryn's story, thereby explaining some of the variability in the experiments and published reports.

Care must also be exercised in interpreting the positive and negative reactions, what is an acceptable background, etc. Suffice it to say that a good deal of preparatory work, standardization, reproducibility, and practice is required before embarking on testing a batch of tissue with immunocytochemical means and rushing to interpret the results for quick publication.

2. Lectin Cytochemistry

Lectins are carbohydrate binding proteins of bacterial, animal, or, most commonly, plant origin. They bear two or more nonimmunological binding sites for sugars. Most lectins bind with the terminal nonreducing sugars of the glycoprotein or glycolipids.[94] The lectins can be conjugated with the fluorescent dyes and the glycoconjugate indirectly visualized the same way as the immunofluorescence. Alternatively, lectins can be biotinylated and then reacted with avidin-horseradish peroxidase conjugate and then visualized in a manner similar to immunoperoxidase techniques. Many commercial kits are now available for easy performance of the lectin binding studies. It has been a trend now whereby the aim of the experiments are shot-gun fishing expeditions to see which of the lectins bind, rather than specific analysis to find out which carbohydrates are altered or expressed. This phenomenon is reflected on the scientific publications which usually report lectin binding property rather than carbohydrate composition. This detour is partly understandable, since the lectins themselves are not absolutely specific either. In any event, quite a lot of valuable information can be gained from such studies. Several studies on lectin binding have been published recently, most pointing to the expression of Gal-β(1→3)-GalNAc as a marker of colorectal cancer and precancer by using peanut agglutinin (PNA).[57,58,61,95] In planning to conduct a study of the carbohydrate marker, the investigative reader is advised to look up the catalogues of the commercial suppliers to consult the list of the various lectins which is constantly being updated yearly if not monthly, and the latest technologies to visualize them.

Essentially, the same general precautions as sounded out under immunocytochemistry also apply to lectin cytochemistry. Which of the two techniques (lectin- vs. immunocytochemistry) is preferable? Orntoft et al.[61] compared the results of lectin binding vs. immunocytochemical detection of Gal-β(1→3)-GalNAc between formalin-fixed and frozen colon tissue; and not unexpectedly, there are differences between the two systems and reactivity to frozen malignant tissue could be demonstrated more often (92%) than the fixed tissue (72%).

3. Enzymatic Detection

Comparative studies of histochemistry and lectin binding have shown that enzymatic (galactose oxidase) oxidation of C-6 hydroxyl groups of galactose and *N*-acetylgalactosamine followed by Schiff's basic fuchsin dye could visualize putative disaccharide residue Gal-β-(1→3)-GalNAc in tracheal gland secretory glycoproteins[96]. Studies in my laboratory comparing the PNA binding and galactose oxidase-Schiff sequence for putative detection of the marker disaccharide Gal-β(1→3)-GalNAc have shown the validity of using this technique in precancer and cancer of the colon.[97] Subsequent studies on a large number of cases from China, Japan, and U.S. show that galactose oxidase-Schiff reactivity can be found in 81.4% of colonic adenocarcinomas, while PNA reactivity is found in 88% of cases.[98] Our studies also reveal that the same polyp, cancer, or the gland within a particular lesion may show differential staining; in other words, while in the vast majority of cases, PNA and galactose oxidase-Schiff reactivity were seen in the same cells, glands, cancers, and polyps, one could have a gland (or polyp or cancer) that is galactose oxidase-Schiff positive and PNA negative and vice versa (Plates 3 and 4, see color plates*).

This discrepancy may indicate our ignorance about the exact nature of the carbohydrate the two techniques are detecting. While the PNA reacts with Gal-β(1→3)-GalNAc, it also binds with the monosaccharide galactose, and further extensive analysis need to be done using the galactose oxidase in order to clearly understand which specific sugar moiety (or moieties) is (are) being detected. In any event, because of the fact that galactose oxidase-Schiff's sequence gives a positive, rather brilliant magenta color in cancer and precancer but not in the normal, we tested its validity in detecting the abnormal mucin in the mucosa remote from carcinoma (Plate 11 of Chapter 5*). A crypt from the apparently normal mucosa (otherwise devoid of dysplastic, atypical, or carcinomatous changes) approximately 5 cm from the tumor margin that shows intense reactivity indicates the presence of the abnormal mucin, in conformity with my field effect theory. Thus, a new test was developed (see Chapter 5).

V. CELL PROLIFERATION

In the colon, the base of the crypt is the site where mitotic activities are normally seen. This area is called the proliferative compartment (PC). Using ³H-thymidine or BrdU incorporation during the DNA synthesis phase, one can measure the rate of DNA synthesis. Alternatively, the mitotic rate can be calculated, albeit a very time-consuming meticulous process. Either of these (the former more preferable because it is less labor intensive) serve as indicators of the rate of cellular proliferation in the crypt and are expressed by the labeling index (L.I., percentage of labeled cells over total cells counted) or percentage mitotic rate (percentage of

---

* See color plates following page 102.

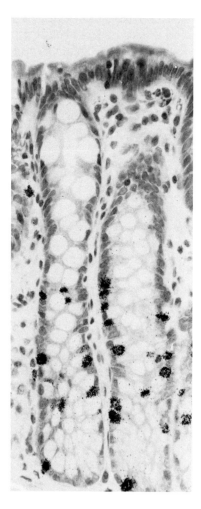 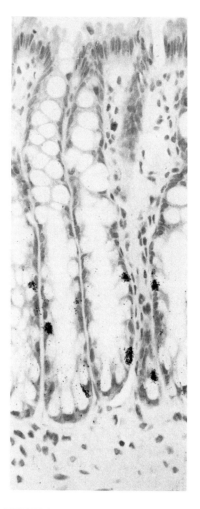

FIGURE 3. ^{3}H-Thymidine autoradiographs of normal colonic crypts showing silver grains localized over a few nuclei, mostly at the lower third to half of the crypts.

FIGURE 4. Autoradiograph of hyperproliferative crypts showing ^{3}H-thymidine labeling in many cells as well as an expansion of the proliferative compartment (compare with Figure 3).

cells undergoing mitosis over total counted). Since cancer is a disorder of uncontrolled cell proliferation, it is therefore natural to look for and find an increased cell proliferation in the colon. In the colon, however, in addition to the increase in these indices, one also sees an expansion of the proliferative compartment (Figures 3 and 4). In support of the field effect theory, investigators working on cell proliferation kinetics have, for quite some time, shown a generalized increase in cell proliferation parameters (increased L.I. and expansion of the PC) of the colonic epithelium in patients with a history of isolated polyps or cancer, familial polyposis, relatives of polyposis patients, etc.[99-105] Because of this generalized increase in cell proliferation parameters, their assay in the rectal mucosal biopsy has been quite popular as a marker in following patients with colorectal cancer undergoing prevention trials. As is the case for all other markers, the influence of appropriate controls (e.g., age matching of subjects, sampling of different areas of the colon, etc.) cannot be over emphasized.[106] Further discussion on the cell proliferation index as an assay for screening or monitoring high-risk individuals is given in Chapter 4.

VI. DNA CONTENT

Another natural curiosity and reward is the fact that during neoplastic transformation, along with increased cell division, one would see aberrant mitoses with aberrant number of chromosomes and perhaps increased DNA in the nuclei of neoplastic cells and those cells that are about to become neoplastic. Using DNA ploidy analysis, it has been demonstrated that the otherwise normal-looking epithelial cells adjacent to and remote from cancer of the colon demonstrate abnormal DNA content, once again in conformity to the field effect.[107-109]

In pilot feasibility studies done on resected colons, mucosal cells were obtained by firmly scraping with a wooden spatula, the spatula then placed in sterile phosphate buffered saline, and vigorously agitated to dislodge the cells.[108] Following homogenization, filtration, and centrifugation, the specimen is fixed in ice cold 70% ethanol. Following RNAse treatment and staining with propridium iodide, the DNA content is measured by flow cytometry.[108] Normal peripheral blood mononuclear cells serve as an internal diploid control.

Ngoi et al.[108] studied the normal-appearing mucosa 2, 5, and 10 cm away from cancer margins in 37 patients with colorectal cancer and reported that the apparently "normal" mucosal cells away from the primary tumor were aneuploid in 48% of cases when the primaries themselves were aneuploid. In addition, cell proliferative activity, as measured by synthetic (S) phase fraction of the aneuploid mucosa (as far away as 10 cm from the tumor margin), was more than double the normal control ($p < 0.0005$).[108]

Thus, it is conceivable that exploitation of this marker and the technology could be rewarding in early detection of cancer in the future.

VII. ONCOGENES AND PRODUCTS

Induction of sarcoma by a virus of chickens by Rous[110] was a milestone in our understanding of the role of small segments of viral genes in cancer formation. Two classes of viruses may cause cancer, the DNA viruses and the retroviruses. The induced cancer may be observed as such in the intact animal *in vivo,* or recognized as transformed cells *in vitro.* The latter is a potpourri of morphological (rounding of cells, piling up of cells that otherwise grow as monolayer) and behavioral changes seen in cells as they are grown in culture dishes (growth of cells in semisolid medium under conditions where normal cells will not grow, immortalization, etc.) and as transplanted xenografts in a suitable host.

Transformation of chicken cells by Rous sarcoma virus (RSV) results in a host of morphological and biochemical changes in the cell, such as disruption of cytoskeletal actin fibers and rearrangement of tubulin, actin, myosin, etc., concomitant with an increased activity of a protein kinase that selectively phosphorylates tyrosine residues. This protein phosphorylating enzyme is of 60-kDa molecular weight and is therefore abbreviated as pp60^{src} since it is the product of a *src* (for sarcoma) gene that causes the sarcoma. Normal vertebrate cells contain the proto-*src* gene which produces pp60 pro-*src* with approximately 1/100th the activity of pp60^{src} of RSV transformed cells. Most acutely transforming RNA viruses contain oncogenic sequences called viral oncogenes (v-*onc*). Over the years, not only have numerous v-*onc* genes been identified, but many normal human cells have also been demonstrated to contain DNA sequences homologous to these v-*onc* genes. These cellular homologues of v-*onc* genes are the so-called c-*onc* or proto-oncogenes. The current dogma is that the viruses have acquired the *onc* gene from the host cells and that the c-*onc* genes are evolutionary progenitors of the v-*onc* genes.[111-113] Our understanding of the relationship between the v-*onc* and c-*onc* genes came about when c-*onc* genes, coupled with retroviral long terminal repeat segments of the

DNA, were transfected (transferred) into quiescent NIH 3T3 cells resulting in their transformation. In addition, when DNA from chemically transformed mouse fibroblasts are transfected to untransformed cells, the latter show evidence of transformation,[114] indicating that genomic sequences could confer transformation to the recipient cells. Similar transforming sequences were demonstrated for human cancers, including those of the colon.[115] The dormant proto-oncogene (or c-*onc*) can be activated by somatic mutation or a retrovirus can acquire the c-*onc* and convert it to an active oncogene. The clues to this phenomenology came from the studies of the oncogene of human bladder carcinoma which is a close homologue of the oncogene acquired by Harvey murine sarcoma virus (v-*ras*[Ha]) from rat genome.[116-118] Another member of the *ras* gene family is the oncogene of Kirsten murine sarcoma virus (v-*ras*[Ki]). The v-*ras* encodes proteins of 21,000 Da (p21) and the different members of the *ras* genes differ by only mutations in codon 12, 13, or 61. A number of studies have addressed the expression of *ras* oncogenes in colorectal cancer where approximately half the cancers were found to express mutated *ras* genes, and there are suggestions that mutation of *ras* proto-oncogenes may be important during colon carcinogenesis in humans.[119-121] Using polymerase chain reaction, Meltzer et al.[122] however concluded that *ras* family proto-oncogene activation is an uncommon event, at least in the precancerous condition of ulcerative colitis. As regards its utility as a marker, immunocytochemical studies in my laboratory have demonstrated the expression of both p21 and mutated p21 in human precancers and cancers.[60] Figures 5 and 6 demonstrate the expression of mutated p21 in the colonic crypts of Crohn's disease and tubular adenomatous polyp.

As mentioned earlier, pp60 is a gene product of Rous sarcoma virus *src*, pp60[c-src] being the cellular homologue of the viral pp60[v-src]. Cartwright et al.[123] recently reported that the protein kinase activity of pp60[c-src] from colonic carcinomas and polyps are increased, indicating activation of c-*src* during colon carcinogenesis. There are reports of increased levels of other oncogenes and products, such as c-*myc* and the gene product p62[c-myc] in colorectal cancer.[124-126]

A conflicting view has recently emerged regarding the p53 gene. While it was initially demonstrated that the product of normal (wild type) p53 gene is necessary for cell growth,[127,128] others consider it to be a tumor suppressor gene since its product suppresses the characteristic growth of transformed cells.[129] Mutation and over-expression of the p53 gene appear to inactivate this growth suppression and has therefore been claimed to be an important event early during colon carcinogenesis.[129] The p53 gene is located in the short arm of chromosome 17 (17p0, a copy of which is lost in a variety of human cancers, including that of the large intestine).[130] Immunocytochemical study with antibodies to p53 demonstrate that a wide variety of tumors, including nearly half of colorectal carcinomas, overexpress the protein.[131,132] What significance these findings has in terms of serving as a marker awaits further investigation.

VIII. ENZYMES AND METABOLITES

A host of different enzymes has been found to be differentially expressed (qualitative or quantitative) in the neoplastic and nonneoplastic colonic epithelium, both in experimental models and in human disease, which may be best looked at under different categories as proposed by Ho et al.,[133] and which I present to you with minor modifications:

A.   Nucleic acid metabolism
        Adenosine deaminase
        Orotate phosphoribosyl transferase
        Cytidine 5′-triphosphate synthetase

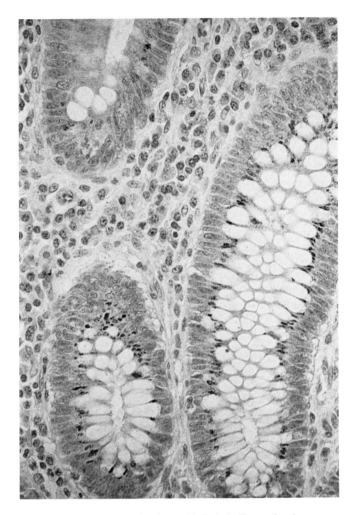

FIGURE 5. Colonic crypts of patients with Crohn's disease showing punctate immunoreactivity with anti-p21^{ser} antibody at supranuclear locations.

Orotidine 5′-monophosphate decarboxylase
Thymidine kinase
Uridine kinase
Uracil phosphoribosyl transferase

B.   Carbohydrate metabolism
Glucose-6-phosphate dehydrogenase
Hexokinase
Lactate dehydrogenase
6-Phosphogluconate dehydrogenase
Pyruvate kinase
Transaldolase

C.   Protein metabolism
Gamma glutamyl transferase
Peptidyl proline hydroxylase

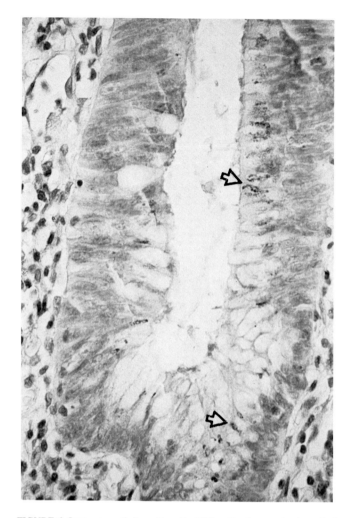

FIGURE 6. Immunoreactivity with anti-p21^{ser} antibody seen in the apical cytoplasm (arrow) of the crypt in a tubular adenomatous polyp.

Phosphoserine phosphatase
Pyrroline-5-carboxylate reductase

D.   Polyamine metabolism
        Ornithine decarboxylase
        S-adenosyl methionine decarboxylase

E.   Miscellaneous
        Aryl sulfatase B
        Urate oxidase
        Plasminogen activator
        Protein kinase C

Of these, only the enzymes of polyamine metabolism, particularly ornithine decarboxylase (ODC) and other isoforms, are being extensively characterized and practically used as markers for identification and monitoring of individuals at high risk of colorectal cancer.[134-137] A recent study by Braverman et al.[138] however, casts some doubt about its potential as a marker.

There are recent interesting reports on enzymes related to signal transduction and cell growth (e.g., protein kinase C, PKC). Study of the experimental colon carcinogenesis in rat indicates an increase in PKC activity following carcinogen administration.[139] Studies of glucose-6-phosphate dehydrogense in patients with adenomatous polyps and ulcerative colitis, and that of adenosine diphosphate ribosyl transferase in mononuclear leukocytes of patients with polyps and cancer, also suggest a differential expression in malignant cells.[140,141] All these studies are preliminary and deserve further investigation and development to validate their usefulness as markers.

IX. MISCELLANEOUS

There are other miscellaneous markers that have been, from time to time, reported to be of use in identifying individuals at high risk. These include measurement of unscheduled DNA synthesis (reduced capacity for mononuclear cell DNA repair synthesis),[142,143] nucleolar organizer region proteins,[144] not to mention the association of skin tags and colon cancer (but not necessarily asymptomatic)![145,146]

X. FIELD EFFECT THEORY

In mid-1976, as a beginner in the area of carcinogenesis and having induced cancer in rats injected with azoxymethane, I was naturally quite excited. This is a phenomenon that some of my readers would probably understand. There were a few tumors in each rat that even I, with my poor eyesight, could appreciate. Being also trained as a pathology resident, I could not help but look at the entire colon under the microscope and, since that was my dissertation project, I did take extra time to look at them! It was evident that a wide variety of progressive changes, both morphological and histochemical, were present throughout the entire large intestine in sporadic fashion. Of course, I rationalized their presence by hypothesizing that the administered carcinogen had acted on the entire epithelium causing multifocal changes throughout the field of action (field effect). Some of these changes were rather early and recognized only as an alteration in mucin phenotype and dilated, distorted crypts, some were more advanced, showing morphological changes that most people are familiar with (atypia/dysplasia, carcinoma), and some were frank carcinomas. I have been trying to find reasons why only a fraction of foci undergo progressive changes. I regret that I have no definite answer; unfortunately, I do not know of anyone else who has! Thanks to the pioneering work of investigators like Berenblum[147] and Pozharisski[6] on the concepts of initiation and promotion, and the significance of cell division on promotion, it is becoming increasingly clear that both DNA damage and cell proliferation are vital to progression of cancer.[148]

Be that as it may, I started to look at the human colon. For obvious moral and ethical reasons, I could not possibly think of such sequential studies of carcinogenesis in the human. So I had to find surrogates that I could use to compare and correlate the events I had observed in these rats. I then rationalized that (1) a patient has colon cancer because of her/his exposure to the carcinogen (a rather elusive item in the human colon, except for the fecapentaenes, see below) and (2) the patient harboring colon cancer would therefore also show progressive changes. I was readily rewarded by the presence of such lesions in the otherwise normal-appearing areas of the colon away from the cancer, as far remote as the distal margin of the surgical resection of the colon (Plate 2, opposite above, see color plates*); these are almost identical to those in the experimental animals. While the recognition of the dilated, distorted crypts and the emergence of sialomucin in the human colon bearing a cancer is nothing new,

* See color plates following page 102.

to equate that they are pre-neoplastic because of their identical appearances is rather radical, and I was aware of the fact that my public disclosure of these would result in public humiliation at the very least. Lawrence Weiss, then a sophomore medical student, wanted to do a required project with me. To be sure that what I was observing is no imagination of mine, I had Larry study the human slides "blindly". It must have been our similarly high myopia; Larry confirmed what I had observed.[7] I had been fortunate to have Benjamin F. Trump as my mentor, who has also been the Chairman of the department; he was quick to accept my observation and interpretation. It was reassuring, as radical as the observation was, I was in no imminent danger of losing my job, at least not on this ground.

My first public presentation was at a National Cancer Institute Small Group meeting on January 25, 1980, organized by my mentors and friends Benjamin Trump and Curtis Harris. Although they did not quite tell me, it might have been a "practice session" before I was sent to the "hungry wolves" in national meetings. Perhaps because most of the audience consisted of rather distinguished scientists working on biochemical aspects of carcinogenesis who could not be too excited about some blue-black mucin change, and there was no G.I. pathologist preoccupied with the polyp-cancer only theory of colon carcinogenesis in the audience, I faced no hostile comment. On the contrary, Gunther Bahr, then at the Armed Forces Institute of Pathology, commented that my findings were interesting, as he had seen such multifocal precancerous changes in human bladder. Glenwood Trivers, in Curtis Harris's laboratory, was more effusive, perhaps because he was not a G.I. pathologist, and discussed at length the implications of such multifocal precancerous changes as a result of field effect of the carcinogen. Glen and I have become very good friends since then; I do not know if his generous support and encouragement at that first meeting with me had anything to do with it, although we rarely ever discussed that particular area of research.

I must admit that this support from a distinguished few and lack of hostility from the majority in the first public presentation of the data gave me all the confidence I ever needed. Then came presentation at national meetings just a month later. In February of 1980, I presented the findings at the International Academy of Pathology Annual Meeting in New Orleans. I was lucky; most in the audience had not rejected my concept and some even thought it had merit. The organizers of the meeting (most notably, Nathan Kauffman) thought that this concept of field effect change in the entire large intestine and the sampling of mucus at the rectum may have great potential in designing future screening tests, and even arranged a press conference. I do not know what that had achieved in terms of the acceptance of the concept by others and advancement of our knowledge and understanding of the problem of early detection and prevention of colorectal cancer. I must emphasize again that the mucin changes had been observed by Filipe and co-workers earlier, but within the rigidity of polyp only-cancer hypothesis, its significance was not understood;[40] with the field effect theory, it appears to make sense.[7]

The results of this study in humans, along with three other papers describing the study in *in vivo* and *in vitro* models were published a year later in the *Journal of National Cancer Institute*. Perhaps out of naivety, I had thought that others would follow up on the concept. Nearly a decade later, my observation of precancerous changes in mucosa remote from carcinoma in the human has been validated by other pathologists;[8] they too were not accepting of the concept of the field-effect of the carcinogen. Curiously, acceptance of my concept came from the use of peanut agglutinin, specific antibody for T antigen,[59,60] cell proliferation kinetics,[102-105,107,108] ornithine decarboxylase assay,[135] DNA ploidy analysis,[108,109] or even morphologically demonstrable changes.[18,108] Orntoft et al.[61] indeed confirmed our observation that the crypts in the mucosa remote from carcinoma that are morphologically subtly abnormal also expressed T antigen. The most confirmatory of all, however, is the fact that the screening test based on this principle does work with greater than 90% sensitivity and specificity (see Chapter 5), along with a more or less similar sensitivity for neoplasm of the different segments of the colon. Had the field effect theory not been operational, one would see a very low sensitivity for neoplasms of the cecum and proximal (right) colon, progressively increasing to the highest level in the rectum. In support of the existence of field effect in other organs, I cannot help but cite a recent paper by Benedetto et al.[149] showing the existence of a biochemical field effect in the human uterine cervix.

In summary, I offer the following rationale, backed by scientific data in support of the field effect theory, and the expected and observed changes in the mucosa remote from a colonic neoplasm:

1. As a result of carcinogen(s) exposure, there are random biochemical alterations in the genome of the colonic epithelial cells throughout the entire large intestine (field effect).
2. In the human, one such carcinogen could be the fecapentaenes, which are present in the feces of people on Western-style diet and appear early in life.[150] Work in my laboratory and elsewhere has demonstrated that the fecapentaenes can cause DNA damage,[151,152] increase cell proliferation in the colon,[151] and even produce tumors,[153,154] albeit extracolonic.
3. The above provides a perfect fit into the model proposed by Cohen and Ellwein,[148] whereby fecapentaene alone, by virtue of causing both DNA damage and cell proliferation, may propagate a few of the initiated cells to cancer. Of course, if there are other reasons for accelerated cell proliferation,[6,155] the cancer would appear early in life and/or in multiple foci, as in ulcerative colitis and Crohn's disease.
4. The so-called "recurrent" cancers at the site of anastomosis of the intestine following resection for a cancer can also be explained. To begin with, as I alluded to in Chapter 2, subsequent cancers can be considered recurrent only if there was histopathological evidence of microscopic carcinoma at the resection margin. In these rare cases, recurrence of cancers takes place within 8 to 22 weeks.[156] In the vast majority of cases where no evidence of overt cancer is seen at the resection margin, there is new cancer formation (metachronous) that appears at a later date, the median time being 18 months.[157] I submit that these metachronous carcinomas are the result of promotion of the initiated foci as a part of the generalized field effect of the carcinogen. The role of uncontrolled and continued carcinogenic stimuli cannot be ruled out either.
5. Where does the polyp fit in? This may be the most difficult one to explain. A recent study by Slater et al.[158] demonstrates that while a synchronous polyp is seen in 30% of patients with a single cancer, 70% of patients with synchronous carcinoma also have synchronous polyp. Does this increased incidence of polyps in conjunction with more than one cancer indicate that the polyps and carcinomas are caused by the same carcinogenic factors, but different, perhaps a higher dose? It is quite possible that, as asserted by the Maskens and Deschner team,[159,160] the polyps are somewhat different biological entities that also become cancer.

REFERENCES

1. **Fenoglio-Preiser, C. M. and Pascal, R. R.,** Other tumors of the large intestine, in *Gastrointestinal and Oesophageal Pathology,* Whitehead, R., Ed. Churchill Livingstone, London, 1989, 747.
2. **Shamsuddin, A. K. M., Bell, H. G., Petrucci, J. V., and Trump, B. F.,** Carcinoma *in situ* and "microinvasive" adenocarcinoma of colon, *Pathol. Res. Pract.,* 167, 374, 1980.
3. **Snover, D. C., Gilbertsen, V. A., and Niratvongs, S.,** Minute adenocarcinoma of the colon arising in flat mucosa: Five cases asking the question: "does *de novo* colon carcinoma exist?", *Lab. Invest.,* 46, 78A, 1982.

4. **Crawford, B. E. and Stromeyer, F. W.,** Small non-polypoid carcinoma of the large intestine, *Cancer,* 51, 1760, 1983.

5. **Shamsuddin, A. M., Kato, Y., Kunishima, N., Sugano, H., and Trump, B.F.,** Carcinoma *in situ* in flat mucosa of large intestine. Report of a case with significance in strategies for early detection, *Cancer,* 56, 2849, 1985.

6. **Pozharisski, K. M.,** The significance of nonspecific injury for colon carcinogensis in rats, *Cancer Res.,* 35, 3824, 1975.

7. **Shamsuddin, A. K. M., Weiss, L., Phelps, P. C., and Trump, B. F.,** Colon epithelium. IV. Human colon carcinogenesis: changes in human colon mucosa adjacent to and remote from carcinomas of the colon, *J. Natl. Cancer Inst.,* 66, 413, 1981.

8. **Lee, Y.-S.,** Background mucosal changes in colorectal carcinomas, *Cancer,* 61, 1563, 1988.

9. **Shamsuddin, A. M., Phelps, P. C., and Trump, B. F.,** Human large intestinal epithelium: light microscopy, histochemistry and ultrastructure, *Hum. Pathol.,* 13, 790, 1982.

10. **Shamsuddin, A. K. M. and Trump, B. F.,** Colon epithelium. II. *In vivo* studies of colon carcinogenesis: light microscopic, histochemical and ultrstructural studies of histogenesis of azoxymethane-induced carcinomas in Fisher 344 rats, *J. Natl. Cancer Inst.,* 66, 389, 1981.

11. **Shamsuddin, A. K. M. and Trump, B. F.,** Colon epithelium. III. *In vitro* studies of colon carcinogenesis in Fischer 344 rats: *N*-Methyl-*N′*-nitro-*N*-nitrosoguanidine-induced changes in colon epithelium in explant culture, *J. Natl. Cancer Inst.,* 66, 401, 1981.

12. **Shamsuddin, A. K. M.,** Morphogenesis of colonic carcinoma-ultrastructural features of azoxymethane-induced early lesions in colon epithelium of Fischer 344 rats, *Arch. Pathol. Lab. Med.,* 106, 140, 1982.

13. **James, J. T., Shamssuddin, A. M., and Trump, B. F.,** A comparative study of the morphological and histochemical changes induced in the large intestine of ICR/Ha and C57Bl/Ha mice by 1,2-dimethylhydrazine, *J. Natl. Cancer Inst.,* 71, 955, 1983.

14. **Shamsuddin A. K. M. and Phillips, R. M.,** Preneoplastic and neoplastic changes in colonic mucosa of Crohn's disease, *Arch. Pathol. Lab. Med.,* 105, 283, 1981.

15. **Shamsuddin, A. K. M., Sugano, H., and Trump, B. F.,** Morphogenesis of large intestinal carcinoma. Its significance in early detection, in *GANN Monograph on Cancer Research,* Vol. 31, Inokuchi, K., Ed., Japan Scientific Societies Press, Tokyo, and Plenum Press, New York, 1986, 59.

16. **McLellan, E. A. and Bird, R .A.,** Specificity study to evaluate induction of aberrant crypts in murine colons, *Cancer Res.,* 48, 6183, 1988.

17. **McLellan, E. A. and Bird, R. A.,** Aberrant crypts: potential preneoplastic lesions in the murine colon, *Cancer Res.,* 48, 6187, 1988.

18. **Roncucci, L., Stamp, D., Medline, A., and Bruce, R.,** Aberrant crypt foci and microadenomas in the human colon, *Am. J. Gastroenterol.,* 85, 1284, 1990.

19. **Pretlow, T. P., O'Riordan, M. A., Kolman, M. F., and Jurcisek, J. A.,** Colonic aberrant crypts in azoxymethane-treated F344 rats have decreased hexosaminidase activity, *Am. J. Pathol.,* 136, 13, 1990.

20. **Heddle, J. A., Blakey, D. H., Duncan, A. M. V., Goldberg, M. T., Newmark, H., Wargovich, M. J., and Bruce, W. R.,** Micronuclei and related nuclear anomalies as a short-term assay for colon carcinogens, in *Indicators of Genetic Exposure,* Banbury Report, Vol. 13, Bridges, B. A., Butterworth, B. E., and Weinstein, I. B., Eds., Cold Spring Harbor, New York, 1982, 367.

21. **Wargovich, M.J., Goldberg, M.T., Newmark, H.L., and Bruce, W.R.,** Nuclear aberration as a short-term test for genotoxicity to the colon: evaluation of nineteen agents in mice, *J. Natl. Cancer Inst.,* 71, 133, 1983.

22. **Seiler, M. W., Reilova-Velez, J., Hickey, W., and Bono, L.,** Ultrastructural markers of large bowel cancer, in *Markers of Colonic Cell Differentiation,* Wolman, S. R. and Mastromarino, A. J., Eds., Progress in Cancer Research and Therapy, Vol. 29, Raven Press, New York, 1984, 51.

23. **Dawson, P. A., Filipe, M. I., and Bussey, H. J.,** Ultrastructural features of colonic epithelium in familial polyposis coli, *Histopathology,* 1, 105, 1977.

24. **Mughal, S. and Filipe, M. I.,** Ultrstructural study of the normal mucosa-adenoma-cancer sequence in the development of familial polypsis coli, *J. Natl. Cancer Inst.,* 60, 753, 1978.

25. **Phelps, P. C., Toker, C., and Trump, B. F.,** Surface ultrastructure of normal, adenomatous, and malignant epithelium from human colon, *SEM/1979/III,* IIT Research Institute, Chicago, 1979, 169.

26. **Riddell, R. H. and Levin, B.,** Ultrastructure of the "transitional" mucosa adjacent to large bowel carcinoma, *Cancer,* 40, 2509, 1977.

27. **Jass, J. R., Filipe, M. I., Abbas, S., Falcon, C. A. J., Wilson, Y., and Lovell, D. A.,** A morphologic and histochemical study of metaplastic polyps of the colorectum, *Cancer,* 53, 510, 1984.

28. **Ansher, A. F., Lewis, J. H., Fleischer, D. E., Cattau, E. L., Jr., Collen, M. J., O'Kieffe, D. A., Korman, L. Y., and Benjamin, S. B.,** Hyperplastic colonic polyps as a marker for adenomatous colonic polyps., *Am. J. Gastroenterol.,* 84, 113, 1989.

29. **Foutch, P. G., Mai, H. D., Disario, J. A., Pardy, K., and Hayden, C. T.,** The sentinel hyperplastic polyp — a marker for synchronous neoplasia in the proximal colon, *Am. J. Gastroenterol.,* 85, 1276, 1990.

30. **Brinkley, B. R. and Chafouleas, J. G.,** Cytoskeleton and the transformed phenotype of malignant cells, in *Markers of Colonic Cell Differentiation,* Wolman, S. R. and Mastromarino, A. J., Eds., Progress in Cancer Research and Therapy, Vol. 29, Raven Press, New York, 1984, 67.

31. **Dudouet, B., Jacob, L., Beuzeboc, P., Magdelenat, H., Robine, S., Chapuis, Y., Christoforv, B., Cremer, G. A., Pouillard, P., Bonnichon, P., Pinnon, F., Salmon, R. J., Pointereau-Bellanger, A., Bellanger, J., Maunoury, M. T., and Louvard, D.,** Presence of villin, a tissue-specific cytoskeletal protein, in sera of patients and an initial clinical evaluation of its value for the diagnosis and follow-up of colorectal cancers, *Cancer Res.,* 50, 438, 1990.

32. **Filipe, M. I.,** The histochemistry of intestinal mucins. Changes in disease, in *Gastrointestinal and Oesophageal Pathology,* Whitehead, R., Ed., Churchill Livingstone, New York, 1989, 65.

33. **Yogeeswaran, G. and Salk, P. L.,** Metastatic potential is positively correlated with cell surface sialylation of cultured murine tumor cell lines, *Science,* 212, 1514, 1981.

34. **Culling, C. F., Reid, P. E., and Dunn, W. L.,** A new histochemical method for the identification and visualization of both side chain acylated and non-acylated sialic acid, *J. Histochem. Cytochem.,* 24, 1225, 1976.

35. **Reid, P. E., Culling, C. F., Ramey, C. W., Dunn, W. L., and Clay, M. G.,** A simple method for the determination of the *O*-acetyl substitution pattern of the sialic acids of colonic epithelial glycoprotein, *Can. J. Biochem.,* 55, 493, 1977.

36. **Reid, P. E., Culling, C. F. A., Dunn, W. L., Ramey, C. W., and Clay, M. G.,** Chemical and histochemical studies of normal and diseased human gastrointestinal tract. I. A comparison between histologically normal colon, colonic tumours, ulcerative colitis and diverticular disease of the colon, *Histochem. J.,* 16, 235, 1984.

37. **Culling, C. F. A, Reid, P. E., and Dunn, W. L.,** A histochemical comparison of the *O*-acylated sialic acids of the epithelial mucins in ulcerative colitis, Crohn's disease and normal controls, *J. Clin. Pathol.,* 32, 1272, 1979.

38. **Muchmore, E. A., Varki, N. M., Fukuda, M., and Varki, A.,** Developmental regulation of sialic acid modifications in rat and human colon, *FASEB J.,* 1, 229, 1987.

39. **Bharathan, S., Moriarty, J., Moody, C. E., and Sherblom, A. P.,** Effect of tunicamycin on sialomucin and natural killer susceptibility of rat mammary tumor ascites cells, *Cancer Res.,* 50, 5250, 1990.

40. **Filipe, M. I. and Branfoot, A. C.,** Abnormal patterns of mucus secretions in apparently normal mucosa of large intestine with carcinoma, *Cancer,* 34, 282, 1974.

41. **Filipe, M. I.,** Mucus secretion in rat colonic mucosa during carcinogenesis induced by dimethylhydrazine. A morphological and histochemical study, *Br. J. Cancer,* 32, 60, 1975.

42. **Bhavanandan, V. P., Katlic, A., Banks, J., Kemper, J. G., and Davidson, E. A.,** Partial characterization of sialoglycopeptides produced by cultured human melanoma cells and melanocytes, *Biochemistry,* 20, 5586, 1981.

43. **Sherblom, A. P., Buck, R. L., and Carraway, K. L.,** Purification of the major glycoproteins of 13762 MAT-B1 and MAT C-1 rat ascites mammary adenocarcinoma cells by density gradient centrifugation by cesium chloride and guanidine hydrochloride, *J. Biol. Chem.,* 255, 783, 1980.

44. **Funakoshi, I. and Yamashina, I.,** Structure of the *O*-glycosidically linked sugar units from plasma membranes of an ascites hepatoma, *J. Biol. Chem.,* 257, 3782, 1982.

45. **Esterly, J. R. and Spicer, S. S.,** Mucin histochemistry of human gall bladder: changes in adenocarcinoma, cystic fibrosis, and cholecystitis, *J. Natl. Cancer Inst.,* 40, 1, 1968.

46. **Bloom, E. J., Itzkowitz, S. H., and Kim, Y. S.,** Carbohydrate tumor markers in colon cancer and polyps, in *Colon Cancer Cells,* Moyer, M. P. and Poste, G. H., Eds., Academic Press, San Diego, 1990, 429.

47. **Itzkowitz, S. H., Yuan, M., Ferrell, L. D., Palekar, A., and Kim, Y. S.,** Cancer-associated alterations of blood group antigen expression in human colorectal polyps, *Cancer Res.,* 46, 5976, 1986.

48. **Itzkowitz, S. H., Yuan, M., Fukushi, Y., Palekar, A., Phelps, P. C., Shamsuddin, A. M., Trump, B. F., Hakomori, S., and Kim, Y. S.,** Lewis^x- and sialylated Lewis^x-related antigen expression in human malignant and nonmalignant colonic tissue, *Cancer Res.,* 46, 2627, 1986.

49. **Yuan, M., Itzkowitz, S. H., Ferrell, L. D., Fukushi, Y., Palekar, A., Hakomori, S., and Kim, Y. S.,** Expression of Le^x and sialylated Le^x antigens in human colorectal polyps, *J. Natl. Cancer Inst.,* 78, 479, 1987.

50. **Yuan, M., Itzkowitz, S. H., Palekar, A., Shamsuddin, A. M., Phelps, P. C., Trump, B. F., and Kim, Y. S.,** Distribution of blood group antigens A,B,H, Lewis^x and Lewis^y in human normal, fetal, and malignant colonic tissue, *Cancer Res.,* 45, 4499, 1985.

51. **Atkinson, B. F., Ernst, C. S., Herlyn, M., Steplewski, Z., Sears, S. F., and Koprowski, H.,** Gastrointestinal cancer-associated antigen in immunoperoxidase assay, *Cancer Res.,* 42, 4820, 1982.

52. **Gong, E., Hirohashi, S., Shimosato, Y., Watanabe, M., Ino, Y., Teshima, S., and Kodaira, S.,** Expression of carbohydrate antigen 19-9 and stage specific embryonic antigen 1 in nontumorous and tumorous epithelia of the human colon and rectum, *J. Natl. Cancer Inst.,* 75, 447, 1985.

53. **Magnani, J. L., Nilsson, B., Brockhaus, M., Zopf, D., Steplewski, Z., Koprowski, H., and Ginsburg, V.,** A monoclonal antibody-defined antigen associated with gastrointestinal cancer is a ganglioside containing

sialylated lacto-*N*-fucopentaose II, *J. Biol. Chem.,* 257, 14365, 1982.

54. **Chia, D., Terasaki, P. I., Suyama, N., Galton, J., Hurota, M., and Katz, P.,** Use of monoclonal antibodies to sialylated Lewis[x] and sialylated Lewis[a] for serological tests of cancer, *Cancer Res.,* 45, 435, 1985.

55. **Kuuselu, P., Jalanko, H., Roberts, P., Sipponen, P., Mecklin, J.-P., Pitkanen, R., and Makela, O.,** Comparison of CA 19-9 and carcinoembryonic antigen (CEA) levels in the serum of patients with colorectal disease, *Br. J. Cancer,* 49, 135, 1984.

56. **Kim, Y. S., Yuan, M., Itzkowitz, S. H., Sun, Q., Kaizu, T., Palekar, A., Trump, B. F., and Hakomori, S.,** Expression of Le[y] and extended Le[y] blood group-related antigens in human malignant, premalignant and nonmalignant colonic tissue, *Cancer Res.,* 46, 5985, 1986.

57. **Boland, C. R., Montgomery, C. K., and Kim, Y. S.,** Alteration in colonic mucin occurring with cellular differentiation and malignant transformation, *Proc. Natl. Acad. Sci. U.S.A.,* 79, 2051, 1982.

58. **Cooper, H. S.,** Peanut lectin-binding sites in large bowel carcinoma, *Lab. Invest.,* 47, 383, 1982.

59. **Elsayed, A. M., Jockle, G., and Shamsuddin, A. M.,** Peanut agglutinin as a marker for preneoplastic and neoplastic changes in human and rat colon, *Proc. Am. Assoc. Cancer Res.,* 27, 201, 1986.

60. **McKenzie, K. J., Purnell, D. M., and Shamsuddin, A. M.,** Expression of carcinoembryonic antigen, T-antigen and oncogene products as markers of neoplastic and preneoplastic colonic mucosa, *Hum. Pathol.,* 18, 1282, 1987.

61. **Orntoft, T. F., Ole Mors, N. P., Eriksen, G., Jacobsen, N. O., and Poulsen, H. S.,** Comparative immunop-eroxidase demonstration of T-antigens in human colorectal carcinomas and morphologically abnormal mucosa, *Cancer Res.,* 45, 447, 1985.

62. **Yuan, M. Itzkowitz, S. H., Boland, C. R., Kim, Y. D., Tomita, J. T., Palekar, A., Bennington, J. L., Trump, B. F., and Kim, Y. S.,** Comparison of T-antigen expression in normal, premalignant, and malignant human colonic tissue using lectin and antibody immunohistochemistry, *Cancer Res.,* 46, 4841, 1986.

63. **Itzkowitz, S. H., Yuan, M., Montgomery, C. K., Kjeldsen, T., Takahashi, H. K., Bigbee, W. L., and Kim, Y. S.,** Expression of Tn, sialosyl-Tn, and T antigens in human colon cancer, *Cancer Res.,* 49,197, 1989.

64. **Springer, G. F., Desai, P. R., and Bawatwala, I.,** Blood group MN specific substances and precursors in normal and malignant human breast tissue, *Naturwissenchaften,* 61, 457, 1974.

65. **Springer, G. F.,** T and Tn, general carcinoma antigens, *Science,* 224, 1198, 1984.

66. **Samuel J., Noujaim, A. A., Maclean, G. D., Suresh, M. R., and Longenecker, B. M.,** Analysis of human tumor associated Thomsen-Friedenreich antigen, *Cancer Res.,* 50, 4801, 1990.

67. **Springer, G. F., Desai, P. R., Tegtmeyer, H., Scanlon, E. F., Fry, W. A., Semerdjian, R. A., and Neybert, C. G.,** Further studies on the detection of early lung and breast carcinoma by T antigen, *Cancer Detect. Prev.,* 8, 95, 1985.

68. **Stein, R., Chen, S., Grossman, W., and Goldenberg, D. M.,** Human lung carcinoma monoclonal antibody specific for the Thomsen-Friedenreich antigen, *Cancer Res.,* 49, 32, 1989.

69. **Limas, C. and Lange, P.,** T-antigen in normal and neoplastic urothelium, *Cancer,* 58, 1236, 1986.

70. **Gold, P. and Freedman, S. O.,** Demonstration of tumor-specific antigens in human colonic carcinomata by immunological tolerance and absorption techniques, *J. Exp. Med.,* 121, 439, 1965.

71. **Wagener, C., Csaszar, H., Totovic, V., and Breuer, H.,** A highly sensitive method for the demonstration of carcinoembryonic antigen in normal and neoplastic colonic tissue, *Histochemistry,* 58, 1, 1978.

72. **Go, V. L., Spencer, R. J., Ravry, M. J., Shorter, R. G., and Huizenga, K. A.,** Carcinoembryonic antigen (CEA) in malignant and inflammatory colonic tissue, *Gastroenterology,* 64, 734, 1973.

73. **Stubbs, R. S., Nadkarni, D. M., and Monsey, H. A.,** Fecal carcinoembryonic antigen (CEA) in patients with large bowel cancer, *Eur. J. Surg. Oncol.,* 13, 433, 1987.

74. **Shively, J. E. and Beatty, J. D.,** CEA-related antigens: molecular biology and clinical significance, *Crit. Rev. Oncol. Hematol.,* 2, 355, 1985.

75. **Zhang, H.-.Z, Ordonez, N. Z., Batsakis, J. G., and Chan, J. C.,** Monoclonal antibody recognizing a carcinoembryonic antigen epitope differentially expressed in human colonic carcinoma vs. normal adult colon tissue, *Cancer Res.,* 49, 5766, 1989.

76. **Fucini, C., Tommasi, S. M., Rosi, S., Malatantis, G., Cardona, G., Panichi, S., and Bettini, U.,** Follow up of colorectal cancer resected for cure. An experience with CEA, TPA, CA 19-9 analysis and second-look surgery, *Dis. Colon Rect.,* 30, 273, 1987.

77. **Fletcher, R. H.,** Carcinoembryonic antigen, *Ann. Intern. Med.,* 104, 66, 1986.

78. **Gold, D. V. and Miller, F.,** Comparison of human colonic mucoprotein antigens from normal and neoplastic mucosa, *Cancer Res.,* 38, 3204, 1978.

79. **Gold, D. V.,** Immunoperoxidase localization of colonic mucoprotein antigen in neoplastic tissue, *Cancer Res.,* 41, 767, 1981.

80. **Pant, K. D., Dahlman, H. L., and Goldenberg, D. M.,** A putatively new antigen (CSAp) associated with gastrointestinal and ovarian neoplasia, *Immunol. Commun.,* 6, 411, 1977.

81. **Pant, K. D., Dahlman, H. L., and Goldenberg, D. M.,** Further characterization of CSAp, an antigen associated with gastrointestinal and ovarian tumors, *Cancer,* 42, 1626, 1978.

82. **Gold, D. V., Nocera, M. A., Stephens, R., and Goldenberg, D. M.,** Murine monoclonal antibodies to colon-specific antigen p, *Cancer Res., 50*, 6405, 1990.

83. **Muraro, R., Wunderlich, D., Thor, A.,Cunningham, R., Noguchi, P., and Schlom, J.,** Immunological characterization of a novel human colon-associated antigen (CAA) by monoclonal antibody, *Int. J. Cancer, 39, 34*, 1987.

84. **Gold, D. V., Ishizaki, G., Keller, P., and Lew, K.,** Generation of a monoclonal antibody (G9) reactive with an organ-specific, tumor-associated epitope of human colon carcinoma, *Cancer Res., 49*, 6412, 1989.

85. **Bara, J., Paul-Gardais, A., Loisillier, F., and Burtin, P.,** Isolation of a sulfated glycopeptidic antigen from human gastric tumors: its localization in normal and cancerous gastrointestinal tissues, *Int. J. Cancer., 21,* 133, 1978.

86. **Bara, J., Loisillier, F., and Burtin, P.,** Antigens of gastric and intestinal mucous cells in human colonic tumors, *Br. J. Cancer, 41*, 209, 1980.

87. **Bara, J., Languille, O., Gendron, M. C., Daher, N., Martin, E., and Burtin, P.,** Immunohistological study of precancerous mucus modification in human distal colonic polyps, *Cancer Res., 43*, 3885, 1983.

88. **Decaens, C., Bara, J., Rosa, B., Daher, N., and Burtin, P.,** Early oncofetal antigenic modifications during rat colonic carcinogenesis, *Cancer Res., 43*, 355, 1983.

89. **Zottner, St., Lossnitzer, A., Hageman, Ph. C., Delemarre, J. F. M., Hilkens, J., and Hilgers, J.,** Immunohistochemical localization of the epithelial marker MAM-6 in invasive malignancies and highly dysplastic adenomas of the large intestine, *Lab Invest., 57*, 193, 1987.

90. **Nuti, M., Teramoto, Y. A., Marani-Constantin, R., Horan-Hand, P., Colcher, D., and Schlom, J. A.,** A monoclonal antibody (B72.3) defines patterns of a novel tumor associated antigen in human mammary carcinoma cell populations, *Int. J. Cancer., 29*, 539, 1982.

91. **Johnson, V. G., Schlom, J., Paterson, A. J., Bennett, J., Magnani, J. L., and Colcher, D.,** Analysis of a human tumor-associated glycoprotein (TAG-72) identified by monoclonal antibody B72.3, *Cancer Res., 46*, 850, 1986.

92. **Paterson, A. J., Schlom, J., Sears, N. F., Bennett, J., and Colcher, D.,** A radioimmunoassay for the detection of a human tumor-associated glycoprotein (TAG-72) using monoclonal antibody B72.3, *Int. J. Cancer, 37*, 659, 1986.

93. **McDowell, E. M. and Trump, B. F.,** Histological fixative suitable for diagnostic light and electron microscopy, *Arch. Pathol. Lab. Med., 100*, 405, 1976.

94. **Damjanov, I.,** Lectin cytochemistry and histochemistry, *Lab. Invest., 57*, 5, 1987.

95. **Caldero, J., Campo, E., Vinas, J., and Cardesa, A.,** Lectin-binding sites in neoplastic and non-neoplastic colonic mucosa of 1,2-dimethylhydrazine-treated rats, *Lab. Invest., 61*, 670, 1989.

96. **Schulte, B. A. and Spicer, S. S.,** Light microscopic histochemical detection of sugar residues in secretory glycoproteins of rodent and human tracheal glands with lectin-horseradish peroxidase conjugates and the galactose oxidase-schiff sequence, *J. Histochem. Cytochem., 31*, 391, 1983.

97. **Elsayed, A. M. and Shamsuddin, A.,** Detection of altered glycoconjugate in preneoplastic and neoplastic human large intestinal epithelia by galactose oxidase-Schiff sequence, *Lab. Invest., 56*, 221, 1987.

98. **Xu, H., Sakamoto, K., and Shamsuddin, A.,** Detection of colonic tumor marker Gal-GalNAc by galactose oxidase-Schiff sequence, *Proc. Am. Assoc. Cancer Res., 32*, 165, 1991.

99. **Deschner, E. E., Lewis, C. M., and Lipkin, M.,** *In vitro* study of human epithelial cells. I. Atypical zone of H^3-Thymidine incorporation in mucosa of multiple polyposis, *J. Clin. Invest., 42*, 1922, 1963.

100. **Deschner, E. E., Lipkin, M., and Solomon, C.,** *In vitro* study of human epithelial cells. II. H^3-Thymidine incorporation into polyps and adjacent mucosa, *J. Natl. Cancer Inst., 36*, 849, 1966.

101. **Cole, J. W. and McKalen, A.,** Studies on the morphogenesis of adenomatous polyps in the human colon, *Cancer, 16*, 998, 1963.

102. **Deschner, E. E. and Lipkin, M.,** Proliferative patterns in colonic mucosa in familial polyposis, *Cancer, 35*, 413, 1975.

103. **Maskens, A. P. and Deschner, E. E.,** Tritiated thymidine incorporation into epithelial cells of normal-appearing colorectal mucosa of cancer patients, *J. Natl. Cancer Inst., 58*, 1221, 1977.

104. **Bleiberg, H., Buyse, M., and Galand, P.,** Cell kinetic indicators of premalignant stages of colorectal cancer, *Cancer, 56*, 124, 1985.

105. **Terpstra, O. T., van Blankenstein, M., Dees, J., and Eilers, G. A. M.,** Abnormal pattern of cell proliferation in the entire colonic mucosa of patients with colon adenoma or cancer, *Gastroenterology, 92*, 704, 1987.

106. **Roncucci, L., Ponz de Leon, M., Scalmati, A., Malagoli, G., Pratissoli, S., Perini, M., and Chahin, N. J.,** The influence of age on colonic epithelial cell proliferation, *Cancer, 62*, 2373, 1988.

107. **Staiano-Coico, L., Wong, R., Ngoi, S. S., Jacobson, I., Morrissey, K. P., Lesser, M. L., Gareen, I. F., McMahon, C., Cennerazzo, W., and DeCosse, J. J.,** DNA content of rectal scrapings from individuals at low and high risk for the development of colorectal cancer, a feasibility study, *Cancer, 64*, 2579, 1989.

108. **Ngoi, S. S., Staiano-Coico, L., Godwin, T. A., Wong, R. J., and DeCosse, J. J.,** Abnormal DNA ploidy and proliferative patterns in superficial colonic epithelium adjacent to colorectal cancer, *Cancer, 66*, 953, 1990.

109. **Bibbo, M., Michelassi, F., Bartels, P. H., Dytch, H., Bania, C., Lerma, E., and Montag, A. G.,** Karyometric features in normal-appearing glands adjacent to human colonic adenocarcinoma, *Cancer Res.,* 50, 147, 1990.

110. **Rous, P.,** A sarcoma of the fowl transmisible by an agent separable from the tumor cells, *J. Exp. Med.,* 13, 397, 1911.

111. **Duesberg, P. H.,** Retroviral transforming genes in normal cells?, *Nature (London),* 304, 219, 1983.

112. **Bishop, J. M.,** Enemies within: the genesis of retrovirus oncogenes, *Cell,* 23,5, 1981.

113. **Slamon, D. J., deKernion, J. B., Verma, I. M., and Cline, M. J.,** Expression of cellular oncogenes in human malignancies, *Science,* 224, 256, 1984.

114. **Shih, C. and Weinberg, R. A.,** Isolation of a transforming sequence from a human bladder carcinoma cell line, *Cell,* 29, 161, 1982.

115. **Cooper, G. M.,** Cellular transforming genes, *Science,* 218, 801, 1982.

116. **Der, C., Krontiris, T., and Cooper, G. M.,** Transforming genes of human bladder and lung carcinomas are homologous to the *ras* genes of Harvey and Kirsten sarcoma viruses, *Proc. Natl. Acad. Sci. U.S.A.,* 79, 3637, 1982.

117. **Parada, L. F., Tabin, C. J., Shih, C., and Weinberg, R. A.,** Human EJ bladder carcinoma oncogene is homologue of Harvey sarcoma virus *ras* gene, *Nature (London),* 297, 474, 1982.

118. **Santos, E., Tronick, S. R., Aaronson, S. A., Pulciani, S., and Barbacid, M.,** T24 human bladder carcinoma oncogene is an activated form of the normal human homologue of BALB- and Harvey-MSV transforming genes, *Nature (London),* 298, 343, 1982.

119. **Bos, J. L., Fearon, E. R., Hamilton, S. R., Verlaan-de Vries, M., Van Boom. J. H., Van der Eb, A. J., and Vogelstein, B.,** Prevalence of *ras* mutations in human colorectal cancers, *Nature (London),* 327, 293, 1987.

120. **Forrester, K., Almoguera, C., Han, K., Grizzle, W. E., and Perucho, M.,** Detection of high incidence of K-*ras* oncogenes during human carcinogenesis, *Nature (London),* 327, 298, 1987.

121. **Vogelstein, B., Fearon, E. R., Hamilton, S. R., Kern, S. E., Preisinger, A. C., Leppert, M., Nakamura, Y., Whyte, R., Smits, A. M. M., and Bos, J. L.,** Genetic alterations during colorectal tumor development, *N. Engl. J. Med.,* 319, 525, 1988.

122. **Meltzer, S. J., Mane, S. M., Wood, P. K., Resau, J. H., Newkirk, C., Terzakis, J. A., Korelitz, B. I., Weinstein, W. M., and Needleman, S. W.,** Activation of c-Ki-*ras* in human gastrointestinal dysplasias determined by direct sequencing of polymerase chain reaction products, *Cancer Res.,* 50, 3627, 1990.

123. **Cartwright, C. A., Meisler, A. I., and Eckhart, W.,** Activation of the pp60$^{c\text{-}src}$ protein kinase is an early event in colon carcinogenesis, *Proc. Natl. Acad. Sci. U.S.A.,* 87, 558, 1990.

124. **Sikora, K., Chan, S., Evan, G., Gabra, H., Markham, N., Stewart. J., and Watson, J.,** c-*myc* oncogene expression in colorectal cancer, *Cancer,* 59, 1289, 1987.

125. **Ciclitira, P. J., Macartney, J. C., and Evan, G.,** Expression of c-*myc* in nonmalignant and premalignant gastrointestinal disorders, *J. Pathol.,* 151,293, 1987.

126. **Stewart, J., Evan, G., Watson, J., and Sikora, A.,** Detection of the c-*myc* oncogene product in colonic polyps and carcinomas, *Br. J. Cancer,* 49,681, 1986.

127. **Mercer, W. E., Avignolo, C., and Baserga, R.,** Role of the p53 protein in cell proliferation as studied by microinjection of monoclonal antibodies, *Mol. Cell Biol.,* 4, 276, 1984.

128. **Shohat, O., Greenberg, M., Reisman, D., Oren, M., and Rotter, V.,** Inhibition of cell growth mediated by plasmids encoding p53 anti-sense, *Oncogene,* 1, 277, 1987.

129. **Baker, S. J., Markowitz, S., Fearon, E. R., Willson, J. K. V., and Vogelstein, B.,** Suppression of human colorectal carcinoma cells growth by wild-type p53. *Science,* 249, 912, 1990.

130. **Fearon, E. R., Hamilton, S. R., and Vogelstein, B.,** Clonal analysis of human colorectal tumors, *Science,* 238, 193, 1987.

131. **Rodrigues, N. R., Rowan, A., Smith, M. E. F., Kerr, I. B., Bodmer, W. F., Gannon, J. V., and Lane, D. P.,** p53 mutations in colorectal cancer, *Proc. Natl. Acad. Sci. U.S.A.,* 87, 558, 1990.

132. **Nigro, J. M., Baker, S. J., Preisinger, A. C., Jessup, J. M., Hostetter, R., Cleary, K., Bigner, S. H., Davidson, M., Baylin, S., Devilee, P., Glover, T., Collins, F. S., Weston, A., Modali, R., Harris, C. C., and Vogelstein, B.,** Mutations in the *p53* gene occur in diverse human tumour types, *Nature (London),* 342, 705, 1989.

133. **Ho, S. B., Toribara, N. W., Bresalier, R. S., and Kim, Y. S.,** Biochemical and other markers of colon cancer, *Gastroenterol. Clinics N.A.,* 17, 811, 1988.

134. **Luk, G. D. and Baylin, S. B.,** Ornithine decarboxylase as a biologic marker in familial colonic polyposis, *N. Engl. J. Med.,* 311, 80, 1984.

135. **Luk, G. D., Desai, T. K., Bull, A. W., Kinzie, J. L., Thompson, R. R., Silverman, A. L., and Moshier, J.,** Rectal mucosal ornithine decarboxylase activity as a marker for colonic polyps and cancer, *Gastroenterology,* 94, A272, 1988.

136. **Hietala, O. A., Yum, K. Y., Pilon, J., O'Donnell, K., Holroyde, C. P., Kline, I., Reichard, G. A., Litwin, S., Gilmour, S. K., and O'Brien, T. G.,** Properties of ornithine decarboxylase in human colorectal adenocarcinomas, *Cancer Res.,* 50, 2088, 1990.

137. **Luk, G. D., Desai, T. K., Conteas, C. N., Moshier, J. A., and Silverman, A. L.,** Biochemical markers in colorectal cancer: diagnostic and therapeutic implications, *Gastroenterol. Clinics N. A.,* 17, 931, 1988.

138. **Braverman, D. Z., Stankiewicz, H., Goldstein, R., Patz, J. K., Morali, G. A., and Jacobsohn, W. Z.,** Ornithine decarboxylase: an unreliable marker for the identification of population groups at risk for colonic neoplasia, *Am. J. Gastroenterol.,* 85, 723, 1990.

139. **Baum, C. L., Wali, R. K., Sitrin, M. D., Bolt, M. J. G., and Brasitus, T. A.,** 1,2-Dimethylhydrazine-induced alterations in protein kinase C activity in the rat preneoplastic colon, *Cancer Res.,* 50, 3915, 1990.

140. **Markowitz, M. M., Johnson, D. B., Pero, R. W., Winawer, S. J., and Miller, D. G.,** Effects of cumene hydroperoxide on adenosine diphosphate ribosyl transferase in mononuclear leucocytes of patients with adenomatous polyps in the colon, *Carcinogenesis,* 9,349, 1988.

141. **Best, A. J., Das, P. K., Patel, H. R. H., and van Noorden, C. J. F.,** Quantitative cytochemical detection of malignant and potentially malignant cells in the colon, *Cancer Res.,* 50, 5112, 1990.

142. **Pero, R. W., Miller, D. G., Lipkin, M., Markowitz, M. M., Gupta, S., Winawer, S. J., Enker, W., and Good, R.,** Reduced capacity for DNA repair synthesis in patients with or genetically predisposed to colorectal cancer, *J. Natl. Cancer Inst.,* 70, 867, 1983.

143. **Pero, R. W., Ritchie, M., Winawer, S., Markowitz, M. M., and Miller, D. G.,** Unscheduled DNA synthesis in mononuclear leucocytes from patients with colorectal polyps, *Cancer Res.,* 45, 3388, 1985.

144. **Ofner, D., Totsch, M., Sandbichler, P., Hallbrucker, C., Margreiter, R., Mikuz, G., and Schmid, K. W.,** Silver stained nucleolar organizer region proteins (Ag-NORs) as a predictor of prognosis in colonic cancer, *J. Pathol.,* 162, 43, 1990.

145. **Graffeo, M., Cesari, P., Buffoli, A., Salmi, A., and Paterlini, Ə.,** Skin tags: markers for colonic polyps?, *J. Am. Acad. Dermatol.,* 21, 1029, 189.

146. **Piette, A. M., Meduri, B., Fritsch, J., Fermanian, J., and Piette, J. C.,** Do skin tags constitute a marker for colonic polyps? A prospective study of 100 asymtomatic patients and metaanalysis of the literature, *Gastroenterology,* 95, 1127, 1988.

147. **Berenblum, I.,** The mechanism of carcinogenesis: a study of the significance of cocarcinogenic action and related phenomena, *Cancer Res.,* 1, 807, 1941.

148. **Cohen, S. M. and Ellwein, L. B.,** Cell proliferation in carcinogenesis, *Science,* 249, 1007, 1990.

149. **Benedetto, C., Bajardi, F., Ghiringhello, B., Marozio, L., Nohammer, G., Phitakpraiwan, P., Rojanapo, W., Schauenstqein, W., and Slater, T. F.,** Quantitative measurements of the changes in protein thiols in cervical intraepithelial neoplasia and carcinoma of the human uterine cervix provide evidence for the existance of biochemical field effect, *Cancer Res.,* 50, 6663, 1990.

150. **Block, J. B., Dietrich, M. F., Leake, R., Laidlaw, S. A., Vinton, N. E., and Kopple, J. D.,** Fecapentaene excretion: aspects of excretion in newborn infants, children, and adult normal subjects and in adults maintained on total parental nutrition, *Am. J. Clin. Nutr.,* 51, 698, 1990.

151. **Hinzman, M. J., Novotny, C., Ullah, A., and Shamsuddin, A. M.,** Fecal mutagen fecapentaene-12 damages mammalian colon epithelial DNA, *Carcinogenesis,* 8, 1475, 1987.

152. **Shioya, M., Wakabayashi, K., Yamashita, K., Nagao, M., and Sugimura, T.,** Formation of 8-hydroxydeoxyguanosine in DNA treated with fecapentaene-12 and -14, *Mutation Res.,* 225, 91, 1989.

153. **Shamsuddin, A. M. and Ullah, A.,** Carcinogenicity studies of fecapentaene-12 in F-344 rats, *Proc. Am. Assoc. Cancer Res.,* 31, 87, 1990.

154. **Weisburger, J. H., Jones, R. C., Wang, C.-X., Backlund, J.-Y. C., Williams, G. M., Kingston, D. G. I., Van Tassell, R. L., Keyes, R. F., Wilkins, T. D., deWit, P.P., van der Steeg, M., and van der Gen, A.,** Carcinogenicity tests of fecapentaene-12 in mice and rats, *Cancer Lett.,* 49, 89, 1990.

155. **Barthold, S. W.,** The role of nonspecific injury in colon carcinogenesis, in *Experimental Colon Carcinogenesis,* Autrup, H. and Williams, G. M., Eds., CRC Press, Boca Raton, FL, 1983, 185.

156. **Eisenberg, S. B., Kraybill, W. G., and Lopez, M. J.,** Long-term results of surgical resection of locally advanced colorectal carcinoma, *Surgery,* 108, 779, 1990.

157. **Michelassi, F., Vannucci, L., Ayala, J. J., Chappel, R., Goldberg, R., and Block, G. E.,** Local recurrence after curative resection of colorectal adenocarcinoma, *Surgery,* 108, 787, 1990.

158. **Slater, G., Aufses, A. H., Jr., and Szporn, A.,** Synchronous carcinoma of the colon and rectum, *Surg. Gyn. Obstet.,* 171, 283, 1990.

159. **Maskens, A. P. and Dujardin-Lotis, R.,** Experimental adenomas and carcinomas of the large intestine behave as distinct entities: most cearcinomas arise *de novo* in flat mucosa, *Cancer,* 47, 81, 1981.

160. **Deschner, E. E. and Maskens, A. P.,** Significance of the labelling index and labelling distribution as kinetic parameters in colorectal mucosa of cancer patients and DMH treated animals, *Cancer,* 50, 1136, 1982.

Chapter 4

CURRENTLY USED OR RECOMMENDED ASSAYS

I. INTRODUCTION

Assays can be used either for diagnosis or for mass screening of colon cancer for early detection. As discussed in Chapter 1, those that are to be used for mass screening have to meet certain basic criteria for them to be cost effective, not only for individual subjects, but also to the society as a whole. Inasmuch as the society bears the brunt due to mortality and morbidity of its members, the society is also financially responsible for alleviating the suffering of its members. Thus, the population-based screening tests must be simple, accurate, inexpensive, noninvasive, must not be uncomfortable, and must have high compliance. Unfortunately, many of the assays that are currently available and at some point or other have been recommended by various groups to be used for screening do not fulfill most of the above criteria. Nevertheless, it is the seriousness of prevalence, incidence, and the associated mortality and morbidity of cancer of the large intestine that prompts health care professionals to recommend any of these tests in spite of their shortcomings. In this regard, most health care professionals tend not to draw a very clear distinction between cost-effective diagnostic tests and screening tests.

Sharing the same concern, the American Cancer Society recommends the following:[1]

1. "Men and women over the age of 40 should have a digital rectal examination every year.
2. Men and women over the age of 50 should have a stool blood test every year.
3. Men and women over the age of 50 should have a sigmoidoscopic examination every three to five years after two initial negative examinations one year apart."

The above recommendations have been made for all asymptomatic individuals; in other words, they are for mass screening of the population. It would be readily apparent for anyone even remotely informed of the financial and procedural aspects of these that some of the procedures for the assays are neither comfortable nor inexpensive, much less simple.

Individuals with a personal history of polyps or cancer of the large intestine, family history of cancer of the large intestine, or inflammatory bowel diseases who are at a high risk of developing cancer are not to be screened; however, they are to be immediately referred for medical attention for close surveillance.

The American Cancer Society makes its recommendation probably with the least bit of bias; however, the same may not be said for those made by various specialty groups such as endoscopists recommending routine colonoscopic examinations, radiologists advocating barium enema, etc.

II. FECAL OCCULT BLOOD TESTS

The fecal occult blood tests (FOBTs) are the most common of all the assays for the detection of colorectal cancer and are based on the following: it is estimated that up to 2.5 ml of blood may be normally lost in stool per day. In abnormal conditions of the gastrointestinal tract such as ulcers, diverticulitis, colitis, anal fissure and hemorrhoids, etc., more than 3 ml of blood may be lost in the stool per day. It is also assumed that neoplasms in the large intestine (cancer or polyp) will shed blood that may not be obvious by the naked eye (hence, the "occult"). Although this assumption is unscientific and fails to recognize the complexity of carcinogenesis or that blood is not a valid marker of precancer and cancer, a variety of different techniques for the detection of blood in stool have been developed over the years. They are collectively called the fecal occult blood tests (FOBT). The first of these tests was based on the discovery that a natural resin extracted from the wood of *Guaiacum officinale,* the gum guaiac, can detect occult blood. This know-how to detect occult blood in stool has been in documented use since 1864,[2] and was proposed for use in detecting gastrointestinal malignancies as early as 1901.[3] Realizing the seriousness of the problem of cancer of the large intestine and the alarming rate at which asymptomatic cancer patients were being missed, Greegor[4,5] used the FOBT for screening over half a century later. In spite of the very poor performance (discussed later) in the absence of better markers and tests, the fact remains that over the years the test has detected many asymptomatic cancers and adenomas, albeit at a very high health-care cost to society and often as chance or serendipity.[6]

A. GUAIAC TEST

The currently popular methods of identification of FOB involve the use of the leuco-dyes, which are colorless compounds that become colored by oxidation. Of these leuco-dyes, guaiac has been used most commonly and several different test kits are available in the market under different names (e.g., Colo-Rect®, Coloscreen®, Fecatest®, or Fecatwin Sensitive®, Haemoscreen®, HemaChek®, Hemoccult®, Quick-Cult®, etc.). Essentially, the ingredients of most of the available kits are similar and contain a specially prepared filter paper impregnated with guaiac and a container with hydrogen peroxide. Because of the similarity of most of these assays with each other and the limitation of space, it is not practical to describe each of them marketed throughout the world; rather, only a few assays will be discussed in detail. The currently popular Hemoccult® (SmithKline Diagnostics, San Jose, CA) provides:

1. Hemoccult® Slides, which are test cards containing natural guaiac resin in standardized paper, and
2. Hemoccult® Developer, a stabilized mixture of less than 5% hydrogen peroxide and 75% denatured ethyl alcohol in aqueous solution

The assay is designed to provide the result within 5 min. The guaiac tests are qualitative assays for the determination of blood based on the oxidation of the phenol in guaiac to a blue-colored quinone (Plate 5, see color plates*); this oxidation reaction is facilitated by peroxidases (in red blood cells), hydrogen peroxide being the substrate of the enzyme peroxidase liberating the nascent oxygen atom.

$$H_2O_2 + Hgb \text{ (or peroxidase)} \quad \rightarrow \quad H_2O + O_2 \text{ (nascent)}$$
$$O_2 + \text{dye (unoxidized, colorless)} \quad \rightarrow \quad \text{oxidized dye (colored)}$$

Hemoglobin, myoglobin, catalases, cytochromes, iron, etc. can also catalyze such oxidation reactions. Therefore, any dietary substance with high peroxidase activity, oxidative agents such as iodide contained in Iodex, Betadine, etc. or drugs that result in microscopic bleeding in the gastrointestinal tract (aspirin, indomethacin, etc.) will and do interfere with the test results. Obviously, food items containing high concentrations of peroxidases (e.g., broccoli, turnips, rare red meat, cantaloupe, cauliflower, red radish, parsnip, artichoke, bean sprouts, etc.) are to be abstained from prior to and during the assay period. Besides these, substances such as myoglobin from animal protein (red meat) could not be distinguished from hemoglobin by the guaiac test, thereby giving a false positive reaction.

There are other limitations of the guaiac tests.[7] Stability of the test result (color reaction) is also a problem. A strong guaiac reaction may remain positive for 7 to 10 d, however, weak

---

* See color plates following page 102.

TABLE 1
Special Diagnostic Diet for FOB

Food and drug	To eat	To avoid
Rare red meat (beef, lamb)		+
Well-cooked fish, poultry, pork	+	
High fiber food	+	
Raw fruits and vegetables		−
Cooked fruits and vegetables	+	
Aspirin and other NSAID[a]		+

[a] Nonsteroidal antiinflammatory drugs, avoid for 7 d prior to and during the test.

eactions fade and may become negative after 2 to 3 d. In order to circumvent this problem of conversion from weak positive to negative reaction, an additional step of rehydration of the filter paper has been incorporated. This however renders the test even more inaccurate by increasing the false positive rate. The asthetically unpleasant practice of collecting one's stool specimen is also a drawback.

While many of the substances discussed above do give a false positive chemical reaction, there are a host of other factors that would suppress the chemical reaction, yielding a false negative result. These include alcohol, antacids, penicillamine, vitamin C, etc. Storage of the feces may also result in a false negative reaction.

The most serious problem, however, has been the very low sensitivity and specificity for large intestinal neoplasm. This issue is discussed later in this chapter.

B. NONGUAIAC TESTS

Besides the guaiac, other dyes have been used in some newer kits; these include orthotolidine (Hematest®) and tetramethylbenzidine (EZ Detect™and Hemo-Fec®). They are all qualitative and their principle is essentially the same. Some of these kits are also available as over-the-counter items in the drug store and offer a certain attractiveness over the others; EZ Detect™ offers the advantage of being aesthetically more acceptable to practice (Plate 6, see color plates*).

Another qualitative test for detection of FOB utilizes the specificity of antigen-antibody reaction (immunochemical assay), allowing specific detection of human hemoglobin and thereby eliminating the cross reactivity with various peroxidase containing food stuff or animal heme. There are several immunochemical assays available. The HemeSelect™ (SmithKline Diagnostics, San Jose, CA) is based on the principle of reverse-passive hemagglutination.[8] It utilizes fixed chicken erythrocytes coated with anti-human hemoglobin antibody which agglutinate in the presence of human hemoglobin in feces. This assay is much more sensitive than the Hemoccult® test, in detecting lesser amounts of blood in the feces.

The HemeSelect™ Fecal Occult Blood Reagent Kit is used in conjunction with the HemeSelect™ Sample Collection Kits. The reagent kit, good for 40 determinations, contains the following:

1. Specimen Diluent (0.15M phosphate buffered saline, pH 7.25 with 0.15% sodium azide as a preservative)
2. Antibody-Coated Cells (lyophilized rabbit anti-human hemoglobin-coated chicken erythrocytes)
3. Hb Positive Control (lyophilized human hemoglobin)
4. Microtiter plate with "U" bottom wells
5. Droppers (25-µl capacity)

* See color plates following page 102.

The Sample Collection Kit and the following are needed:

1. Pointed-tip forceps
2. Pipettes (0.5 and 0.6 ml capacity) for reconstituting lyophilized reagents
3. Microtiter plate cover
4. Timer for timing the incubation period
5. 0.5% Sodium hypochlorite
6. Adjustable pipette with disposable tips (50 to 200 µl capacity)

Additional materials and equipment needed for proper conduction of the assay include microtiter plate mixer (automatic rotary shaker), microtiter plate viewer, containers for collecting stool specimens, 37°C incubator for drying the microtiter plates, and detergents for washing the microtiter plates.

Since the test is not based on the peroxidase activity of red blood cells, certain dietary restrictions of the guaiac-based tests do not apply. Patients are however recommended to be on a high residue diet commencing 2 d prior to and through the test period (3 consecutive or closely spaced bowel movements). Aspirin and other NSAIDs and alcohol, that may cause gastrointestinal tract irritation and bleeding, are to be similarly abstained from.

Considerable care has to be given in preparation of the reagents and the stool samples for obtaining accurate test results. The lyophilized antibody-coated cells and the human hemoglobin positive control are to be reconstituted 30 min prior to testing; once reconstituted, they should be stored at 2 to 10°C and used within 14 d. The stool sample is to be applied uniformly on the Sample Collection Cards and two of the paper disks with thin and uniform layer of the stool specimen are to be placed in the microtiter wells containing the specimen diluent. These steps are then followed (Plate 7, see color plates*):

1. Extract as much specimen as possible from the disk
2. The samples are diluted and aliquoted
3. Add reconstituted antibody-coated erythrocytes and mix
4. Incubate at room temperature (15 to 30°C) for not less than 30 min
5. Since the hemagglutination patterns are stable for 60 min after completion of incubation, the result is to be read within this period (Plate 8, see color plates*).

Labsystems Oy (Helsinki, Finland) provides a kit that contains 2 assay systems (Figure 1): the guaiac-based, first-step screening assay is the Fecatwin Sensitive® and the second assay is the immunological FECA-EIA which reduces the false positive rate of the former.[9] The Fecatwin Sensitive® provides a chromatography paper that is impregnated with guaiac resin and tightly sealed in a plastic case. Two small disks can be removed from this kit for use in the FECA-EIA. The FECA-EIA is an indirect solid-phase immuno-assay[10] that conveniently utilizes the fecal fluid eluted from the EIA disks of the first-step Fecatwin Sensitive® kit. Anti-human hemoglobin antibody (Ab) is attached to the polystyrene surface of cuvettes which would specifically bind with the hemoglobin antigen (Ag); following washing, alkaline phosphatase-conjugated anti-human hemoglobin antibody (AbE) is added to form a sandwich reaction. After washing to remove the excess enzyme conjugated antibody, the substrate *p*-nitrophenyl phosphate (pNPP) is added, which is converted to yellow-colored *p*-nitrophenol and is read using a spectrophotometer at 405 nm.

1. Ab + Ag
2. Ab + Ag + AbE (Ag sandwiched by two Abs)
3. Ab + Ag + AbE + pNPP → read absorbance at 405 nm.

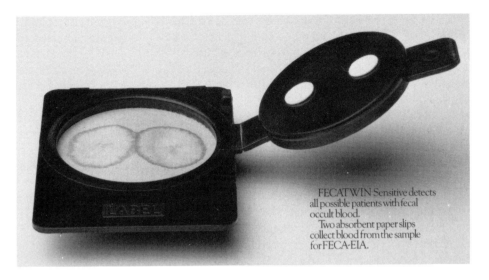

FIGURE 1. FECA-EIA Test kit containing the reagents for first step Fecatwin Sensitive® and immunoassay. Courtesy of Marja-Liisa Huhtala, Ph.D., Labsystems Oy, Helsinki, Finland.

In a study involving 10,343 subjects[9] with 66.5% (6878) participation, Fecatwin Sensitive® was positive in 54% (3719) of the cases. When these subjects underwent further testing by the second-step FECA-EIA, 340 individuals were scored positive (above an absorbance of 0.4 OD at 405 nm). Some 118 cases were further evaluated by endoscopy to reveal 7 (5.9%) cases of adenocarcinoma and 44 (37.3%) cases of neoplastic polyps. Clearly, this study shows that the combination of the second-step immunoassay reduces the false positive rate. Hakkinen et al.[9] contends that by setting the lower limit of positivity to 0.8 OD for absorbance at 405 nm, the false positive rate could perhaps be reduced without substantially increasing the false negative rate.

Besides the complexity of the reactions, cumbersome preparation of specimen and reagents, requirement of spectrophotometers, etc., these techniques also suffer from the high cost and the length of time to perform. The assays still suffer from the inability to detect degraded blood; therefore, the proximal colonic neoplasms are more likely to be missed.

As opposed to these, a quantitative yet sensitive, 90-min assay had been introduced for FOB called HemoQuant® (SmithKline BioScience, Van Nuys, CA). The test is based on the removal of iron from the normally nonfluorescent heme (iron-protoporphyrin complex) of hemoglobin, resulting in the liberation of free porphyrin which is intensely fluorescent and assaying the intensity of fluorescence.[11]

$$\text{Fe-Protoporphyrin complex} \quad \rightarrow \quad \text{Free Porphyrin} \quad + \quad \text{Free Fe}$$
$$\text{(nonfluorescent heme of Hgb)} \qquad \text{(highly fluorescent)}$$

The advantage of HemoQuant® is that it detects both upper and lower gastrointestinal tract bleeding with similar sensitivity since the reaction process is valid for both the intact heme and the one that might have been degraded during transit through the intestinal tract. The assay can only be done in a laboratory and not in the physician's office or clinic settings, and must therefore be sent to the reference laboratory. Automated methods have been developed at the Mayo Clinic, allowing assays of 100 to 150 samples per h.[11] Although the performance of this assay is superior to the guaiac-based ones, the delay (up to a week) in obtaining the result from the reference laboratory makes the physician somewhat less enthusiastic about this assay.

Besides this, the wisdom of using blood itself as a marker of large intestinal neoplasia and the utility of the numerous assays, all detecting blood is now being seriously addressed, to the credit of the original developers of the tests[12,13] and others,[6,14-16] to cite a few. Although initially a sensitivity of 97% was reached for colorectal cancer by the HemoQuant® test, subsequent quantitative determinations of FOB show that fecal blood levels are commonly normal in patients with asymptomatic colon cancer.[12]

As can be gathered from the preceeding, patient education and prior preparation is vital in conducting FOBTs. A total of six tests (two samples from each of three consecutive stools) are to be performed, unless any of the prior tests is a positive one.[7] Thus, the patient should abstain from the interfering substances not only for 3 to 7 d prior to the beginning of sampling, but must continue with those restrictions through the testing period until all the tests (up to six) are performed. These restrictions (Special Diagnostic Diet) include the avoidance of rare red meat, high peroxidase-containing food (*vide supra*), vitamin C, iron tablets, etc. for at least 48 h prior to and during the test period. Aspirin and other nonsteroidal anti-inflammatory drugs (NSAID) are to be avoided for 7 d prior to and during the test period. A delay of more than 6 d between preparation of the stool sample and testing may result in a false negative reaction.

Depending on the individual test kit, the manufacturer's recommendations must be followed. However, the public does not necessarily adhere to the recommendations, be they by the physicians or the manufacturers; anecdotal stories of stool sampling from toilet basin by cooking pans (!) are rather familiar. As regards these restrictions and aesthetic limitations, EZ Detect™ is claimed to be advantageous, given the limitation of not using certain bowl cleansers.

C. PERFORMANCE

The sensitivity and specificity of the FOBTs span a wide range; besides the investigator's bias,[12] some of the discrepancy may be explained by the use of different study designs, patient population, and the extent of follow-up. Another important factor is the confirmation of the mass lesions by the so-called gold standard *viz.* colonoscopy. The outcome of colonoscopic examination depends not only on the extent of colonoscopy, but also on the training and expertise of the colonoscopist. Many a colonoscopist does not examine the entire large intestine up to the cecum and, therefore, to the very least, 33% of the neoplasms may be missed by simply not examining past the sigmoid. In a study of 88 asymptomatic subjects undergoing colonoscopy to the cecum, Johnson et al.[18] found 24 neoplasms in 22 patients; 11 of the 24 neoplasms were in the right (5) and transverse (6) colon. Alarmingly, the FOBTs were negative in 21 of the 22 patients with neoplasms (95.5% false negative rate), only 1 of 6 stool samples from the single positive patient was reactive for FOB. Be that as it may, and not to be distracted from the moral of the story, it is of paramount importance not only in validating the result of any screening test but also for providing adequate health care, to examine the entire length of the large intestine (cecum included) by colonoscopy.

After being in use for nearly 3 decades, the performance of FOBTs is now being critically evaluated.[12-16] As stated at the beginning of the chapter, the purpose of screening tests is early detection of cancer or precancer in asymptomatic individuals. If the patients diagnosed to have cancer were clinically symptomatic and were also positive for FOBTs, it is a coincidence. Indeed, recent critical evaluations point to this chance association and serendipity.[6] However, despite these arguments, the poor sensitivity and specificity of these assays, and the failure of FOBTs to reduce the colon cancer mortality[11] in the absence of better markers and tests (until recently), recommendations for the use of FOBTs continues.[17]

How many asymptomatic cancers or polyps have been detected by FOBTs? The bleak report by Johnson et al.[18] is, unfortunately, not an isolated one, only 1 of 47 patients diagnosed of colon cancer had FOBT positivity as the sole presenting feature,[19] an extreme example of the insensitivity of FOBTs (2.1% sensitivity)! Another extreme example is the 95.7% false positive rate reported by Winchester et al.[20] The sensitivity for the precancerous polyps is worse than the cancers.[16] While, in general, the sensitivity and specificity of guaiac-based FOBTs has been less than 10 and 40%,[16] respectively, there are other published reports claiming up to 80% sensitivity and specificity, albeit for the nonguaiac-based, more accurate and cumbersome immunological test[21] and HemoQuant®.[12]

It cannot be overemphasized that the performance or lack thereof of the FOBTs are not necessarily due to the limitation of the tests themselves; rather, they reflect upon the faulty and unscientific premise of blood as the marker of cancer or precancer of the large intestine. Ahlquist et al.[12] demonstrated that in a selected group of cancer patients, the mean hemoglobin level was 3.3 mg/g stool as measured by HemoQuant®; 38% of these patients were within the normal range (<2 mg Hgb/g stool) for HemoQuant® and 70% patients were Hemoccult® negative. Besides, many conditions of the gastrointestinal tract may cause bleeding and many substances, as noted above, can interfere with the test, resulting in improvization of the technology. But alas, most if not all of those improvements have been for better detection of the "marker" blood. Thus, over the years, the newer technologies have been better detectors of blood in stool (high sensitivity for hemoglobin), yet the improvement in sensitivity and specificity of the assays for cancer and precancerous lesions have not been proportionate, either to the cost of the assays or the investment in terms of human resources and capital worldwide. A case in point is the vast difference between the accuracy in determination of FOB by the qualitative Hemoccult® and the quantitative HemoQuant® test.[12]

Since the original publication by Greegor[4] nearly a quarter of a century ago, FOBTs have been fairly widely used throughout the world. Inasmuch as they have helped save a good many lives from premature death (at a high health care cost to the society), the debate continues to be on the cost effectiveness for using them as screening tests.[12-21] It is to be pointed out that, to the best of my knowledge, none of these FOBTs has been approved by the governmental regulatory agencies (such as the U.S. Food and Drug Administration) for cancer screening; rather, their approval has been for the detection of blood in stool. Indeed, the product instructions themselves claim their utility for detecting occult blood, often with disclaimers that they are not tests for colorectal cancer or any other specific diseases. Fortunately or unfortunately, in reality the tests are being used for screening of populations for cancer or polyp of the large intestine. If one takes into account the recommendations of the American Cancer Society[1] (*vide supra*) and the yield of the positive reaction of FOBTs, an estimated 3 million asymptomatic Americans would have to undergo further testing by barium enema, colonoscopy etc. at an estimated cost of nearly $2.5 billion. If the estimation of the population at risk is taken into account, nearly 6 million Americans who are alive today will die of cancer of the colon or rectum,[22] thereby doubling the above estimated cost. One therefore cannot be overcritical about the cost effectiveness of mass screening tests. It is one more reason to look for accurate and reliable assays.

III. CARCINOEMBRYONIC ANTIGEN (CEA)

Carcinoembryonic antigen, believed to be a cancer-specific antigen, was first isolated from carcinomas of the colon in 1965 by Gold and Freedman.[23] It is a glycoprotein antigen, expressed by both cancer, and fetal and embryonic gut tissue during the first two trimesters of gestational age; hence, it is named carcinoembryonic antigen or CEA. Other markers have also been identified that show a similar common expression and are called oncofetal markers. Although initially it was considered to be a specific marker for colon cancer, CEA has however been demonstrated to be expressed not only in large intestinal cancer, but also in normal and inflammatory lesions of the intestine.[24,25] Given the fact that cancer of the large intestine was (and still is) a major public health concern and there were no other scientifically credible markers and expression of CEA by the colorectal tumor tissue that looked promising, an assay was developed to measure it in the serum.[26] Two major categories of assays are now available for the determination of serum CEA, *viz.* radioimmunoassay[27,28] (RIA) and enzyme-linked immunosorbent assay[29] (ELISA). They are both based on the principle of competitive affinity of binding between the antigen and the antibody molecules.

Simply put, given a fixed number of antibody, only a similar number of antigen (say, CEA) will bind to the antibody. If none or very little CEA is present in the reaction mixture, then the antibody will remain unreacted or only some of them will be reacting to the antigen and others remain free. Both assays utilize this phenomenon of competitive binding; in the radioimmunoassay, one of the components is radiolabeled, so that it is possible to quantitate the free vs. the reacted antibody. A parallel standard assay is run using known amounts of the antigen, and the unknown amount in the sample is quantitated by comparison with the standard. In spite of the highly specific nature of RIA, it suffers from the drawbacks associated with the storage, handling, disposal, potential health hazard, and the limited shelf-life of the isotopes.

In the ELISA system, an enzyme replaces the isotopic label of the RIA. The enzyme is conjugated or tagged to the antigen or the antibody, and the antigen-antibody reaction is quantitatively determined by measuring the activity of the enzyme on the appropriate substrate. The antigen-antibody reaction is amplified by the enzyme activity. The separation of enzyme-labeled immunoreactant which has participated in the antigen-antibody reaction from that which has not, can be done by various techniques such as centrifugation, immunoprecipitation, or binding one of the components on to a solid phase. A reactant which participates in an antigen-antibody reaction can be separated from that which has not, by simply washing the solid phase with the buffer solution. Various solid phases such as polyacrylamide beads, filter papers, etc. are available. To date, the 96-well plastic microtiter plates are, however, the most convenient of all. Figure 2 shows a schematic diagram of the principle of ELISA.

The ABBOTT CEA-EIA One-Step (Abbott Laboratories, North Chicago, IL) is a noncompetitive ELISA that uses the Guinea pig antibody (Ab) as the solid-phase reactant (anti-CEA antibody coated on beads). In a sandwich-type reaction similar to that described under FECA-EIA, the sample containing CEA, the antigen (Ag) is incubated for 2 h along with horseradish peroxidase-conjugated mouse anti-CEA antibody (AbE). Both the immobilized antibody (from Guinea pig) and the enzyme-labeled antibody (from mouse) bind to CEA like a "sandwich". Following removal of unbound materials by washing the beads, the enzyme substrate *o*-phenylenediamine (OPD) is added with hydrogen peroxide. The enzyme reaction is stopped by addition of 1 N sulfuric acid and the reaction product, a yellow-orange color is then quantitated by spectrophotometric absorbance at 492 nm.

1.   Ab on beads + CEA
2.   Ab on beads + CEA + Ab with enzyme (sandwich)
3.   Ab on beads + CEA + Ab with enzyme + OPD + H_2O_2
4.   Measure yellow-orange reaction product at 492 nm.

Testing of unknown patient sample, known standards, and control are performed at the same time. A standard curve, plotting the CEA concentration (on the horizontal or X axis) vs. the mean of absorbance at 492 nm (on the vertical or Y axis), is generated from a set of known duplicate standards (Figure 2). The concentration of CEA in the patient sample is then determined by comparing its mean absorbance (plotted on Y axis) and the corresponding CEA value from the X axis. Figure 3 shows a typical standard curve and the data as printed out for an assay.

A newer procedure called IMx™ (Abbott Laboratories, Abbott Park, IL), which includes a microparticle enzyme immunoassay (MEIA) and a fluorescence polarization immunoassay

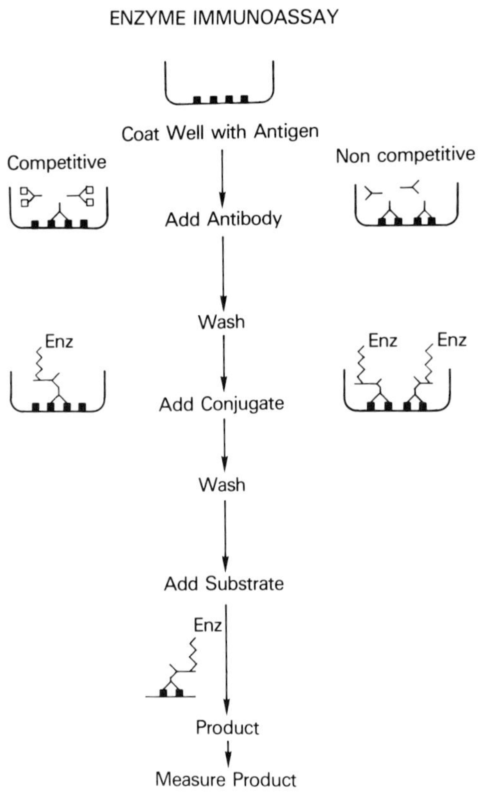

ENZYME IMMUNOASSAY

FIGURE 2. Principle of ELISA. The wells of the microtiter plate are coated with either the antigen or the antibody. In this diagram, the wells are coated with the antigen (solid box). Increasing dilutions of antibodies are added along with the sample which may contain the antigen in question (e.g., CEA depicted as open box). This allows for a competition (left panel) between the antigen in the fluid phase (that is free in the sample) and the antigen in the solid phase (bound to the wells) for reacting with the antibody (depicted as Y). Each set of wells (usually 3 to 4) contain a different, but known dilution of antibody but a constant amount of antigen in the solid phase. If there is more fluid-phase antigen in the sample, the antigen-antibody reaction will be in its favor and few antibodies will bind to the solid-phase antigen. Washing will remove the antigen-antibody complex in the fluid-phase, leaving only a few antibodies bound to the solid-phase antigen. Addition of an enzyme-conjugated antibody against the first antibody followed by substrate reaction will show little reaction which would be indicative of a large amount of antigen in the sample. Alternatively, if there are few or no fluid-phase antigens in the sample, the antibodies will bind to the solid-phase antigen, will withstand washing, and subsequent reactions with the enzyme-linked antibody against the primary antibody will show high activity indicative of low or no antigen in the sample. A parallel standard reaction is done with increasing or decreasing (known) amounts of antigen in the fluid phase to generate a standard curve. The unknown sample is tested in the same manner and its values are quantitated by calculating the degree of antigen-antibody reaction (or inhibition) as it corresponds to the data points in the standard curve. The noncompetitive assay (used in the current assays for CEA) is depicted on the right side. Here the sample is added directly to the solid-phase reactant, followed by an enzyme-conjugated antibody.

(FPIA), is now available which can determine the CEA values in shorter time period than the one described above. The technology uses microparticles (submicron size) coated with a "capture" molecule that specifically binds with the CEA. After incubation of the microparticle and the sample, the reaction mixture is transferred to an inert glass fiber matrix to which the microparticles bind in an irreversible manner. Instead of the horseradish peroxidase, the enzyme used here is alkaline phosphatase and the substrate is a fluorescent compound (methylumbelliferyl phosphate; the fluorescent product of enzyme activity reflecting the antigen-

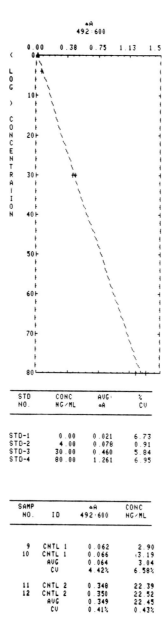

STD NO.	CONC NG/ML	AVG ⌃A	% CV
STD-1	0.00	0.021	6.73
STD-2	4.00	0.078	0.91
STD-3	30.00	0.460	5.84
STD-4	80.00	1.261	6.95

SAMP NO.	ID	⌃A 492:600	CONC NG/ML
9	CNTL 1	0.062	2.90
10	CNTL 1	0.066	⟨3.19
	AVG	0.064	3.04
	CV	4.42%	6.58%
11	CNTL 2	0.348	22.39
12	CNTL 2	0.350	22.52
	AVG	0.349	22.45
	CV	0.41%	0.43%

FIGURE 3. A standard curve generated during the performance of CEA assay showing concentration of CEA in one axis and the absorbance in the other. Courtesy of Janet S. Kilpatrick, B.S., M.T.(ASCP), Clinical Immunology Laboratory, University of Maryland Hospital, Baltimore, MD.

antibody reaction is measured at 448 nm). Similar to the previous assay, the standard curve is generated and the unknown values are estimated by comparison, the MEIA Optical Assembly can automatically determine all these.

CEA immunoreactivity can be determined in the plasma, as can a variety of extravascular body fluids such as, saliva, gastro-duodenal, biliary and pancreatic juices, ascites, pleural effusions, urine, spinal fluid, cyst fluids, etc. The CEA assays are, however, usually performed on plasma. Because of the nature of the assay procedure (Figure 2), it is recommended that the same commercial test package be used for the same patient, preferably in the same laboratory, to minimize interlaboratory variation of results. In general, a plasma CEA value ≤2.5 ng/ml is considered normal, that greater than 5 ng/ml abnormal and advanced malignancy is to be suspected if it is >20 ng/ml.

Since its discovery, numerous studies have been undertaken to examine the utility of CEA for screening, diagnosing, staging, and monitoring the recurrence of colorectal cancer, prognosis, etc. It was soon found not to be suitable as a screening test for far too many high false positive results. Besides the cancers of various other organs, cigarette smoking, chronic pulmonary disease, inflammatory bowel diseases, pancreatitis, etc. are associated with increased plasma CEA levels and therefore its use has now been limited to post-operative monitoring of the recurrence of colorectal cancer;[30,31] that too, only if the preoperative CEA level was high and the level falls to normal baseline (usually 4 to 6 weeks post-operatively). The patient is to be monitored by subsequent periodic determinations (usually at 2 to 3-month intervals), preferably in the same laboratory; increased values indicate recurrence or metastases. It is however estimated that because of the very high false positive rate of CEA elevations and associated high cost of diagnosis and therapy, there is a high marginal cost effectiveness ratio varying from $22,963 to $4,888,208 per quality adjusted life-year saved![32] Kievit and van de Velde therefore contend that CEA monitoring should not be used for routine follow-up of colon cancer patients.[32]

IV. ENDOSCOPIC EXAMINATIONS

It is interesting to note that around the time when the FOBT was introduced (rather, reintroduced) for early detection of colorectal cancer, there came the endoscopic examination in the late 1960s. The documented attempts for direct visualization of the large intestine, however, started as early as in the late 1920s. Not unexpectedly, it was a radiologist who, in 1928, described his attempt to visualize the colon with a 5-feet-long flexible rubber tube attached to an enema can.[33] Later development of flexible fiber optics was a significant milestone. The fiberoptic endoscope principally consists of a series of glass fibers packed in a tight bundle so that light falling on one end of the bundle is transmitted to the other. Although references to such a technology have been documented as far back as in 1927,[34-35] it was not until the late 1950s that the technology was improved to allow visualization of the stomach.[36-38] The menace of gastric cancer in Japan had led the Japanese investigators to work mostly on that problem, resulting in the development of the gastrocamera. It was therefore natural that such a device or modifications thereof would be tried in the case of the large intestine. In the late 1950s, Matsunaga et al.[39] and later Niwa,[40] reported their attempts to examine the colon with a modified gastrocamera, albeit with not much success. After approximately a decade of problem solving, Niwa et al.[41] from Japan and Overholt[42] from the U.S., reported the successful use of a fiber optic endoscope in visualizing the rectum and the sigmoid colon; interestingly enough, around the same time! These earlier endoscopes were short (35 or 65 cm) and their range is up to the sigmoid colon; hence, they are called sigmoidoscopes. As the experience with inserting the endoscope into the lumen of the large intestine grew, so did the interest and determination to go beyond and explore the entire colon. Soon, longer endoscopes (108 cm) became available, with which the investigator can reach up to the mid or proximal transverse colon.

Hiromi Shinya, working with William Wolff at the Beth Israel Medical Center in New York, designed a snare cautery device consisting of a flexible wire which he introduced through the biopsy channel of the endoscope, and set off a revolutionary process of snare

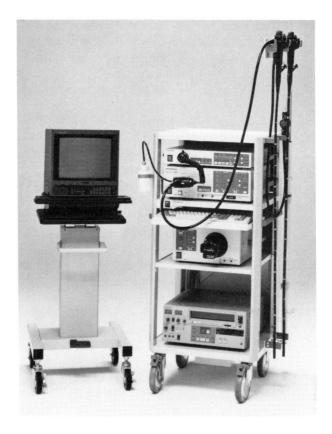

FIGURE 4. An Olympus colonoscopy unit with several colonoscopes
hanging on the right side, video recording device, and monitor.

polypectomy by endoscopy.[43,44] Thus, with a modern day fiber optic colonoscope, it is possible
not only to visualize the large intestine all the way to the cecum and often the terminal ileum,
but also remove small polyps. A typical 168-cm long fiber optic colonoscope, has a pair of
fiber bundles that illuminates the area ahead of the tip of the endoscope. In addition, a channel
for inflating air, a suction channel not only for suction but also for introducing biopsy
instrument, cytology brush or polypectomy snare, and a water injection nozzle to flush clean
the lens are also standard features. The revolution in computer technology has made it possible
not only for the examining physician to visualize, but also the data to be stored and displayed
by video equipment. Figure 4 shows one of the latest models, an Olympus Colonoscopy unit
with CRT monitor and video recording device.

A. PREPARATION

The following criteria are to be met in consideration of successful fiber optic endoscopic
visualization of the colon;[45] (1) the lumen of the large intestine must be meticulously clean so
that fecal debris does not impair the view; (2) the large intestine ahead of the colonoscope tip
must be inflated with air to create a space; (3) for proper visualization, the space must be
lighted and the image has to be transmitted back to the operator; (4) the endoscope tip must
be able to move in the direction of the open lumen (poly-directional tip); and (5) proper
maneuvering by the operator.

The preceding demonstrates that not only the training, experience, and skill of the endoscopist are important, much of his/her ability to visualize is also dependent on the cleanliness
of the intestine and, therefore, the field of examination. Patient preparation is also of paramount importance, which is usually done by having the patient drink a colon lavage solution.

Approximately 2 liters of the lavage solution is administered to the patient at 4 to 6 hours before the examination. The patient usually has several bowel movements as a result of the lavage fluid (containing polyethylene glycol, Na_2SO_4, $NaHCO_3$, NaCl, and KCl dissolved in tap water) and thereafter is ready for examination.

B. PROCEDURE

The patient is usually given an i.v. sedative to help relax and alleviate apprehension and rendering him/her more cooperative. The patient is asked to lie on his/her left side and the fiberscope, attached by a semiflexible sleeve and properly lubricated (Xylocain jelly), is inserted into the anus and then to the rectum. The bowel ahead of the endoscope must be inflated with air and under direct vision; the colonoscope is advanced into the space created by the air. The colonoscope is advanced inch by inch by repeating this maneuver as often as necessary. Once the colonoscope has passed the sigmoid colon, with the sleeve being in the recto-sigmoid area, the colonoscope is "unlocked". This maneuver enables easy handling of the colonoscope and repeat insertion (if necessary) less uncomfortable. The patient is then turned to a supine position and the colonoscope is advanced to the cecum. The colonoscope is slowly pulled backwards inch by inch while closely observing the mucosa and recording the pictures (Plate 9, see color plates*). Patients who have intra-abdominal adhesions or exceptionally tortuous colons pose a problem in navigating the colonoscope. The expert colonoscopist uses several skillful maneuvers (alpha, reverse alpha, pull-back, gamma maneuvers, etc.) to navigate past some of the difficult angles.[45]

C. COMPLICATIONS

As with any other procedure, colonoscopy is also not free of complications. Morbidity from diagnostic colonoscopy is approximately 3 in 1000; the incidence of perforations following polypectomy however can be as high as 1%, which is certainly a serious problem.[45] The pathogenesis of some of these complications are understandable; for instance, a diverticulum could "blow out" as a result of excessive intracolonic air pressure. A large-mouthed diverticulum could be mistaken as the lumen of the intestine and, before long, the tip of the colonoscope could be into the peritoneal space. For that matter, any other condition that would weaken the wall of the large intestine (such as inflammatory bowel diseases, carcinomatous involvement, etc.) could increase the chance for complications of this nature. Certainly, the more skilled the endoscopist, the less is the risk.

D. PERFORMANCE

There has been great debate regarding the usefulness of the colonoscope since the time it was introduced; the debate continues, albeit at a lower, more simmering intensity than at the beginning. Much of the debate is perhaps raised by professional rivalry, fear of losing the "turf" and, the dearest of all, the economics — rather, the politics — of which professional group to be benefited or hurt as a result of this new methodology in health care. Not unexpectedly, many of these criticisms against colonoscopy came from the corners where the radiologists are.[43] While the radiologists would like to claim that their techniques are capable of "doing the job", the endoscopist holds his own ground rather firmly, insisting that their's is the "Gold Standard". The fact that an internal organ can be visualized, samples for further investigation can be obtained, and even polyps can be removed with very little complications, quite justifiably has made this diagnostic procedure a very useful one. No doubt, this technique is to be performed on patients who have abnormal screening test(s), abnormal barium enema examination, or other reasons for referral, including strong family history of colon cancer or previous history of colon cancer, etc.[46] Whether or not colonoscopy should be used as a screening assay is another matter that is certainly to be debated and, with a cost of $423 to $700 for each procedure and the associated discomfort, it will continue to

* See color plates following page 102.

be debatable; in this matter, turf has less to do with it than the economics of the health care cost of the entire nation.[47-49]

A point that has been tangentially made before and cannot be overemphasized is that the performance of any technical test procedure, such as endoscopy, is as good as the training, experience, skill, motivation, and not the least, the mood of the operator. The instrument of choice which, in turn, is determined by the operator's skill, also determines the outcome of the diagnostic procedure. In a comparative study, Ferrands et al.[50] demonstrated that the yield of carcinomas for rigid sigmoidoscopy was a mere 8.8% compared to 79.4% for flexible sigmoidoscopy and 76.5% for double contrast barium enema; the yield of total neoplasms (polyps + cancers) was 11.9%, 90.5%, and 76.2%, respectively. An added issue is the limitation of sigmoidoscopy; Johnson et al.[18] demonstrated what can be easily predicted is that as many as 46% of polyps and cancers could be missed if endoscopy is restricted to the left colon.

V. RADIOLOGICAL EXAMINATIONS

A. BARIUM ENEMA

Based on their experience in detecting cancer with good accuracy, radiologists are increasingly becoming vocal in recommending the barium enema as a cost-effective method for screening large intestinal cancer.[51] Indeed, citing the fact that 10 to 20% of the lesions that are seen radiologically are missed by endoscopy, a rather high false negative rate for a procedure branded as the "gold standard" by the gastroenterologists, the radiologists advocate the use of barium enema for screening. Other arguments in favor of barium enema over colonoscopy are: incomplete visualization of the entire large intestine, a rather high rate of perforation and, of course, the higher cost of endoscopy ($144 to $244 for barium enema vs. $423 to $750 for colonoscopy).[51]

Radiologic visualization of the large intestine however began at the early part of this century. The current techniques utilize either (1) solid-column examination with barium enema alone, or (2) the double-contrast examination by using barium and air. The solid-column examinations are done for patients who are at a low risk of developing cancer or those who are suspected to already have a large enough cancer. The reader would note this is already past the stage of early detection! The double-contrast barium enema is used for patients between the ages of 35 and 75 years of age who are at a high risk of developing cancer of the large intestine. Since the double-contrast (also called air-contrast) barium enema examination better visualizes subtle mucosal abnormalities, this is usually done in patients when small mucosal lesions are suspected[52] (Figure 5).

Like endoscopic examination, radiologic examination also requires fairly elaborate patient preparation, the degree of which varies from center to center and from radiologist to radiologist. They all include prior cleansing of the bowel with laxatives, suppositories or combinations thereof, and abstinence from solid food for about 24 h. There are several contraindications to performing a barium enema examination. First of all, the patient's age and heart condition are two very important factors. Barium enema has precipitated cardiac arrhythmias, even in otherwise healthy individuals. Recent biopsies of the intestine which, as one would easily predict, will carry a high probability of perforation and therefore would be a contraindication for barium enema. Likewise, if there are other diseases of the colon that would enhance the risk of perforation (such as toxic megacolon), these would also be contraindications. Patients who have other serious systemic illnesses likewise, at the discretion of the radiologists, would be contraindicated from undergoing a barium enema examination. The readers would be able to rationalize the reasons for such care from following description of the procedure.

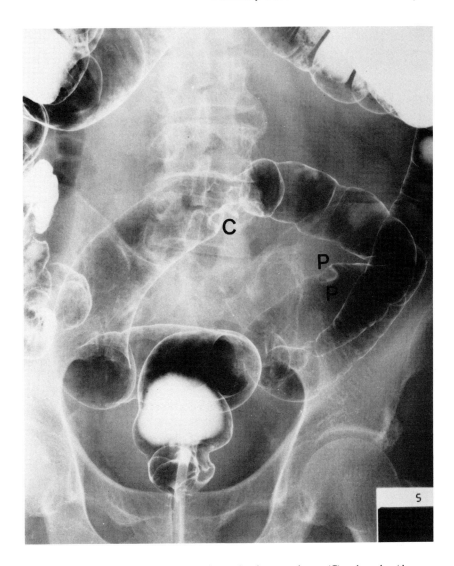

FIGURE 5A. Air-contrast barium enema picture showing a carcinoma (C) and a polyp (the space between the two Ps) in the sigmoid colon.

In preparation for barium enema, a pilot plain film of the abdomen is obtained to ascertain the feasibility of further procedures, for there may exist contraindications, such as evidence of perforation of the colon (free air), toxic dilatation of the colon, etc. Evidence of diverticulitis may alert the radiologist to modify the subsequent procedures a bit. A digital rectal examination is performed which also helps to relax the anal sphincter for the next step of inserting a balloon (optional) enema tip. An i.v. injection of 1 mg glucagon is given to relax the colon (contraindications are pheochromocytoma and insulinoma).

For introducing the barium (a suspension of 20% weight per weight, E-Z-EM Company, Westbury, New York), the patient lays prone while the barium is instilled by hand compression of the bag. Under fluoroscopic visualization, the barium is allowed to traverse the sigmoid and descending colon, up to the splenic flexure, at which time the patient's position is changed to right side down. This position allows the additional help of gravity in moving the barium. Air is insufflated at this time so that it pushes the barium ahead of it to the transverse colon and the hepatic flexure. To bring the barium all the way to the cecum, the patient has to be changed to the supine or upright position. After the barium has reached the cecum, the patient

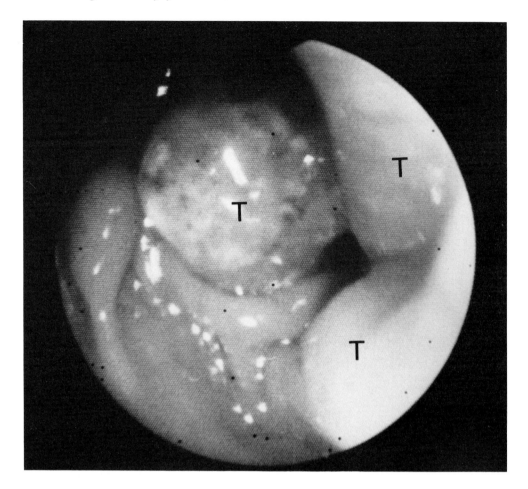

FIGURE 5B. Colonoscopic visualization of the carcinoma identified by the letter T; note that the carcinoma has circumferentially involved the wall of the colon, leaving only a narrow lumen (black rounded space encircled by the tumor). Courtesy of Kosaku Sakamoto, M.D., Gunma University School of Medicine, Maebashi, Japan.

is placed upright and more air is added. Following drainage of the rectal barium and deflation of the balloon, films are taken for evaluation.

Figures 5 through 7 illustrate some examples of colorectal cancer and polyps that have been diagnosed by radiological techniques. Figure 6 shows a filling defect, outlining a carcinoma of the descending colon, and Figure 7 a carcinoma of the sigmoid.

For a barium enema

Sensitivity	76.5%
Specificity	Undetermined
Cost	$144–$244
average	$200
Subject discomfort	Moderate

B. OTHER INDIRECT VISUALIZATIONS

The computerized axial tomography (CAT) scan has been used in conjunction with other diagnostic modalities in colorectal cancer. The cost of such a procedure however limits its application to that of an adjunct methodology, particularly in patients where advanced disease is suspected, such as metastases to distant organs (Figure 8).

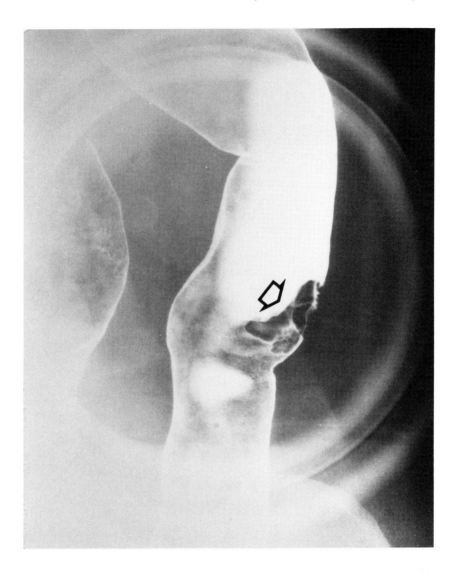

FIGURE 6. Filling defect caused by a carcinoma of the descending colon (arrow) is shown in a 58-year-old patient. Courtesy of Kosaku Sakamoto, M.D., Gunma University School of Medicine, Maebashi, Japan.

VI. MISCELLANEOUS RECOMMENDATIONS

Besides the above popularly used diagnostic and "screening" assays, several other assays have, at one time or another, been proposed to be useful for colorectal cancer detection. These are: cell proliferation kinetics, ornithine decarboxylase, polyamines, methane, etc.

As has been discussed in Chapter 3, the rate and pattern of proliferation of the colonic epithelial cells in the crypt changes during cancer formation. This has been well documented both in numerous experimental models and in human diseases. The altered, rather enhanced cell proliferation can be monitored directly by calculation of mitotic rate, percentage of cells entering into the S phase (DNA synthesis) of cell cycle, etc., or indirectly by measurements of various enzymes and metabolites involved in cell division. Although these indices of cell proliferation discriminate the normal from precancer and cancer (Chapter 3), and are therefore considered to be markers, their use is restricted to the research laboratory for identification and

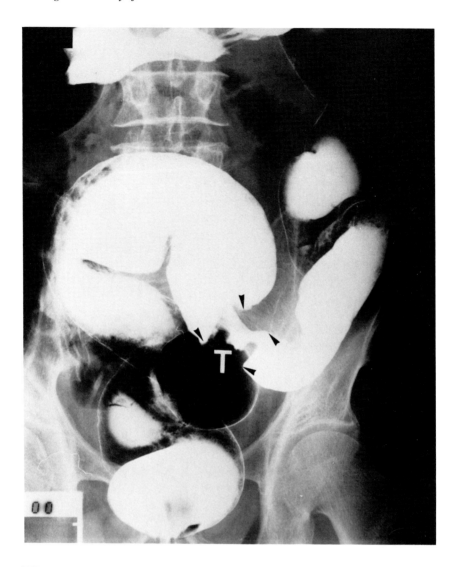

FIGURE 7. An "apple-core" lesion, typical of a carcinoma of the colon is shown. Note that the barium fills the colon and the rounded contour of the colon is preserved on either side of the cancer (T). However, there is an abrupt narrowing of the lumen beginning at the two arrowheads on the left; in the area of the tumor, the intestinal wall is thickened, resulting in an apple-core appearance reflecting the narrow lumen, the contour is regained past the two arrowheads on the right. Courtesy

monitoring of individuals at high risk of colon cancer, monitoring the efficacy of various substances in reducing the risk of colon cancer, etc.[53]

In the subsequent section, particularly dealing with the markers of cell proliferation, I shall frequently refer to normal colon or normal subjects. The reader is reminded that, as discussed in Chapter 2, the definition of normal colon has to be a strict one, one which is free from any known diseases and not the normal-looking epithelium from patients with colon cancer or other diseases.

A. CELL PROLIFERATION KINETICS

The base of the colonic crypt (or gland) is where cell division in the normal colon takes place and therefore serves as the source of new cells and crypts. The cells undergoing mitotic division are found in the lower two-thirds of the crypt (proliferative compartment), mostly in

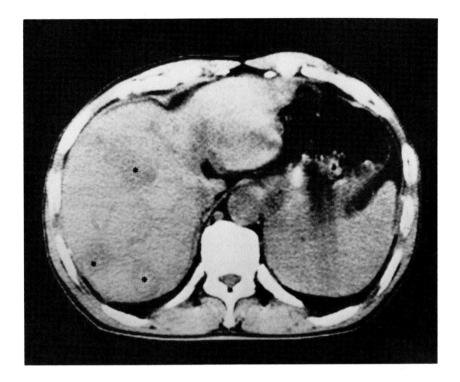

FIGURE 8. CAT-scan picture of the abdomen of the same patient with carcinoma as seen in Figure 7. Several rounded areas of diminished density (darker areas marked by an *) representing metastatic carcinoma are seen in the right lobe of the liver. A larger area, perhaps also representing metastases, is also seen in the left lobe. Courtesy of Kosaku Sakamoto, M.D., Gunma University School of Medicine, Maebashi, Japan.

the lower third, and, to a lesser extent, in the middle third. Early during carcinogenesis, there is both a quantitative and a qualitative change in the proliferative compartment; that is, not only are there more cells undergoing mitosis in the proliferative compartment, but also there is an expansion of the proliferative compartment itself. Besides the mitotic rate, the determination of which is somewhat tedious, the proliferative compartment can also be outlined by labeling the cells undergoing DNA synthesis. The latter can be done either by allowing incorporation of radiolabeled (³H) thymidine deoxy-ribose (³H-TdR) or by a newer method of bromo-deoxy-uridine (BrdU) incorporation by the cells that are actively synthesizing DNA and visualizing the cells by developing the grains from radioactivity (for ³H-TdR) or using immunocytochemical techniques (for BrdU). Which ever way one measures them, the "major zone" of DNA synthesis in the crypt of the normal human or experimental animal is at the lower third of the crypt. The methods of procedure of these are described in subsequent sections.

We owe Deschner and co-workers much of our education and understanding of the subject, and I have therefore taken the liberty of quoting their work extensively, for there is no better way to pay tribute to these pioneers. Deschner outlines the various progressive changes[54] which are observed in the colonic mucosa of patients who are at a high risk of developing colon cancer.[55-60]

Stage I proliferative abnormality is merely an extension of the proliferative compartment (from the lower two-thirds of the crypt) to involve the entire crypt up to the luminal surface.

Stage II proliferative abnormality, on the other hand, is a shift of the "major zone" of DNA synthesis from the normal, lower third to the middle and upper regions of the crypts.

Hyperproliferative crypts with a very high proportion of cells undergoing DNA synthesis and characterized by the above stage I and stage II abnormality express a further stage in the development of neoplasia and are categorized under stage III abnormality.

1. ^{3}H-Thymidine (^{3}H-TdR) Assay

Tiny mucosal biopsy specimens (≤3 mm in diameter) of the colorectal mucosa are incubated in organ culture medium with ^{3}H-TdR (1 μCi/ml) for 1 h. During this time, the culture dishes are usually rocked at 10 cycles per min in an atmosphere of 95% O_2 + 5% CO_2. These tiny mucosal pieces are then carefully embedded in paraffin to ensure proper longitudinal orientation of the crypts, and 5 μm histological sections are cut and mounted on glass slides. Following deparaffinization, by passing through xylene and decreasing concentration of alcohol, the slides are usually treated with Kodak nuclear track material at 45°C. The slides are then dried in dark in a light-tight box with desiccant at 4°C. The duration of this exposure of the beta-rays to the photographic material varies from laboratory to laboratory and also depends on the specific activity of the ^{3}H. Usually, duplicates or triplicates of the control slides are processed and developed at periodic intervals to determine optimum time of exposure. Following development, the slides are lightly stained with hematoxylin and the grains overlying the nucleus of epithelial cells are counted. Background grains on other cells and tissues are estimated, nuclei underlaying more grains than the background are considered labeled, and the labeling index (LI) is calculated by examining a number of cells and crypts sufficient to reach statistical validity and representative of the tissue and disease in question.

$$LI = \frac{\text{Total number of }^3\text{H-TdR labeled cells}}{\text{Total number of epithelial cells counted}} \times 100$$

Figure 3 of Chapter 3 shows an example of the labeling by ^{3}H-TdR in normal and a hyperproliferative crypts. As has been pointed out, it is important that not just the LI be measured, but the expansion or contraction of the proliferative compartment, stage I, II, and III abnormalities, are evaluated.[53,61-63] In order to achieve this, the investigator must therefore divide the crypts into several segments (usually five) and then assess the labeling and/or mitotic rate. The same principle also applies to the BrdU assay.

2. Bromodeoxyuridine (BrdU) Assay

This is a relatively new technique that was introduced in the early 1980s and has quickly found wide acceptance because of its ease, simplicity, and rapidity of assay.[64-67] The principle is very simple; BrdU is a thymidine analogue which is similarly incorporated in to the newly synthesized DNA during the S phase and can be easily visualized by using specific antibody and immunocytochemical techniques.

Similar to the ^{3}H-TdR assay, the colorectal mucosal pieces in explant culture are incubated with BrdU (10^{-4} to 10^{-7} *M),* fixed in formalin, embedded in paraffin, histological sections cut and mounted on chrom alum-coated slides, deparaffinized, and rehydrated with graded ethanols in preparation for immunocytochemistry. The following steps of procedure used in Dr. Elizabeth McDowell's laboratory in our department have produced reproducibly excellent results:

1. Endogenous peroxidase activity is removed with 1% H_2O_2 in absolute methanol at room temperature for 20 min
2. Pepsin digestion (0.4 mg/ml in 0.1 *M* HCl at 37°C for 30 min) removes nonspecific protein binding sites
3. Wash with PBS-Tween 20 (0.5%)
4. DNA hydrolysis in 4 *M* HCl for 20 min (causes single stranded breaks to allow easy access by the antibody)
5. Neutralize with Borax wash for 10 min and wash with PBS.

6. React with mouse anti-BrdU antibody (1:40 in PBS) for 16 to 20 h at room temperature and wash with PBS
7. Incubate with biotinylated anti-mouse IgG (1:200 in PBS) for 30 min at room temperature
8. Incubate with ABC solution (Vector Labs, Burlingame, CA) for 60 min at room temperature and wash with PBS
9. Localize peroxidase with 0.01% DAB solution, rinse slide in chilled tap water, and lightly counterstain slide with hematoxylin
10. Dehydrate in graded ethanols, displace in xylene, mount coverslip, and examine under a microscope

The cells incorporating BrdU are identified by the brown coloration of the DAB precipitate and the results are similar to the ^{3}H-TdR assay and, therefore, ^{3}H-TdR is rapidly being replaced by this new technology. An added advantage is that it is now possible to quantitate the extent of BrdU incorporation by using the optical data digitizer.[67] Welberg et al.[68] recently report that by cutting the colonic explants prior to incubation with BrdU and use of a microwave oven at the beginning of incubation gives excellent results. As one can see from the methods of procedure outlined above, the BrdU technique is much simpler and takes less time. The individual investigator however may wish to modify these steps of procedure to obtain the best result.

3. Scopes and Limitations

Since unrestricted cell division is essential for cancer formation, it is not difficult to understand the rationale for using indices of cell proliferation as assays to determine the risk of cancer and precancer. There are also enough experimental data to support this logical relationship between increased cell proliferation and eventual risk of cancer.[61-63]

A common misconception has been that the LI alone is indicative of the risk of cancer or precancer. A recent study by Lipkin et al.[53] illustrates that LI alone may be deceptive, and that the size and location of the proliferative compartment are more important. Studies in our laboratory on 1, 2-dimethylhydrazine-induced colon cancer in ICR/Ha mouse have shown an expansion of the proliferative zone only in the most susceptible segment of the large intestine.[61] Besides this, insight into the duration of various phases of cell cycle can be studied by the above two techniques. For example, Bleiberg et al.[69] and Terpstra et al.[70] demonstrated that the normal-appearing crypts of patients with adenoma or carcinoma have a longer duration of S phase in addition to a higher LI, in support of mucin changes in this epithelia and the "field effect" theory (Chapter 3).

One should be familiar with the limitations of the measurements of cell proliferation kinetics as assays for colon cancer diagnosis or screening. An important issue is the sampling. It is a well-known fact that, inasmuch as the different regions of the large intestine are morphologically and histochemically different,[71-74] the cell proliferation kinetics are also different, a substantially lower number of proliferating cells in the ascending colon than in the descending colon. This reduced proliferative activity in the ascending colon may, in part, explain the lower rate of cancer in that part of the large intestine.[73-75] The outcome of the assay will also be different for different ages of the subject,[59,60,76] times of day and night of sampling, etc.[77-78] The effect of age is particularly important in this regard since in any study of the population at risk of colon cancer, there would be a wide range of subject age. Roncucci et al.[76] demonstrated that the mean LI of normal individuals of age 66 to 90 years was significantly higher than younger age groups (12.9 vs. 9.5). Analysis of the LI per crypt compartment also showed that there is an expansion of the proliferative zone to the most superficial portion of the crypts; in persons older than 65, the superficial most compartment (of a total of 5) shows consistently and significantly ($p < 0.01$) higher LI than the younger individuals. Interestingly, the LI of these individuals (>65 years old) was almost identical to that of patients with colorectal polyps, who are definitely at a higher risk of colorectal cancer.[76] This study therefore makes at least two very important points: technically speaking, studies of proliferative indices must be done with age-matched controls and both LI and expansion or contraction of the proliferative zone should be evaluated. From an equally important viewpoint of the genesis of cancer, this study demonstrates that individuals at a higher age group (>65 years) are at higher risk of colorectal cancer even if they are free of any known precancerous lesions.

The other limitation is the use of organ culture during the incubation with ³H-TdR or BrdU. It is well known that within the first 48 to 72 h during organ culture, the colonic epithelial cells undergo extensive necrosis and exfoliation;[79,80] what, if any, influence this process may have on a fundamental behavior of cells such as DNA synthesis and cell proliferation remains to be evaluated.

B. ENZYMES AND METABOLITES ASSOCIATED WITH CELL PROLIFERATION

As was discussed in Chapter 3, ornithine decarboxylase (ODC) is a key enzyme in the synthesis of polyamines which are important in cell proliferation. Polyamines (putrescine, spermine, spermidine, cadaverine, etc.) are ubiquitous compounds which are synthesized by a wide variety of cells. The level of ODC is low in normal non-proliferative tissues. However, both ODC and polyamines are elevated in a variety of malignant and rapidly proliferating tissues, including the cancer of the large intestine.[81-85] Similar to the cell proliferation kinetics data supporting my field effect theory of carcinogenesis and marker expression in the colon (Chapter 3), studies of ODC assay in the rectal mucosal biopsy remote from colon cancer also show an increased level, hence serving as a marker with potential for diagnostic assay in precancer and cancer of the large intestine.[86] Besides the use of ODC assay in potential identification of individuals at high risk, it may serve as a monitor in the follow-up of high-risk groups undergoing chemoprevention trials. Although this chapter may not necessarily be the most appropriate forum, I cannot help but mention an intriguing development in this regard. Difluromethylornithine (DFMO) is a selective inhibitor of ODC resulting in rather sustained depletion of polyamines and growth retardation of many cells, including cancer cells both *in vitro* and *in vivo*.[85,87-91] Clinical trials of DFMO and monitoring of its efficacy are ongoing in several centers throughout the world.

ODC has a very short half-life (7 to 15 min) and therefore its assay is "tricky" and extreme care must be given in its assay. ODC has been assayed in the research laboratory by radiochemical and, to a lesser extent, immunohistochemical methods. A flow cytometric method has recently been reported to be a useful one.[92]

1. Radiochemical Assay[82]

The colonic mucosal biopsies are homogenized in 1:10 (wt:vol) of sodium phosphate buffer (100 mM, pH 7.2) containing 5 mM dithiothreitol. An aliquot of mucosal homogenate is reacted to 0.1 mM pyridoxal phosphate and 0.22 mM L-ornithine containing DL-[1-¹⁴C]-ornithine hydrochloride, the cell protein is quantitated by Lowry's method, and the results are expressed as nanomoles of $^{14}CO_2$ released per hour, per milligram of cell protein.

2. Immunohistochemical and Flow Cytometric Assay[92]

Both the immunohistochemical and the flow cytometric methods utilize anti-ODC antibody. The cells are fixed with 2% paraformaldehyde and permeabilized with 0.05% Triton X-100 for 15 min at 4°C. Following washing with PBS, the cells are incubated with anti-ODC antibody applied (1:500, in PBS containing 0.1% gelatin) for 30 min at 4°C. Following washing, FITC conjugated secondary antibody (against the species of the primary anti-ODC antibody) is added. Fluorescence microscopy can be used to visualize the activity and the data can also be collected with an analytic flow cytometer adjusted to an output of 15 mW at 488 nm excitation and 525 nm emission.[92]

The advantage of the new flow cytometric method is that it allows determination of ODC in different subpopulations of cells that may have varying amounts of ODC activity and therefore appears promising as an assay method. In contrast, the radiochemical method determines the total ODC activity and the dilutional effect, if any, of the unwanted tissues or cells (such as submucosal or lamina proprial fibroblast, macrophages, etc.) is not known.

As mentioned above, the ODC assays have some potential utility, at least in a research setting, for identification and monitoring of high-risk individuals. The same cannot be said about the usefulness of polyamine determinations. Studies by Loser et al.[84] suggest that serum or urine polyamine determination has very little utility as a diagnostic assay for colon cancer since a variety of nonmalignant gastrointestinal diseases result in elevated levels. However, similar to the CEA assay, the polyamine levels normalize following curative operations and are further elevated in patients with metastases or relapse; thus, they may have some utility in monitoring the prognosis and recurrence of the disease.[84]

C. SONOGRAPHY

Conventional sonography does not allow adequate assessment of the large intestine because of the presence of gas within the lumen. However, by instilling fluid into the colon, Limberg[93] has been successful in diagnosing colorectal cancers and polyps with rather high sensitivity and specificity and advocates the use of sonography in the diagnosis and perhaps screening. As in barium enema and endoscopy, prior preparation of the bowel is a necessity which consists of 3×10 g magnesium sulfate laxative 24 h before the examination or a lavage on the morning of examination. An injection of 20 mg *n*-butyl-scopolamine-bromide is then given, followed by instillation of up to 1500 ml of water. Scopolamine is given to achieve maximum relaxation and distension of the colon filled with water. It also suppresses the sense of urgency for bowel evacuation as a result of distension. From the time of water instillation, continuous transabdominal sonographic examination of the large intestine is done with a real-time scanning device (5-MHz sector or convex array), with the patient lying on a manual tilting table. At the beginning of sonography, the patient should be in an oblique position so as to distend the recto-sigmoid area, 300 to 400 ml of water is first instilled. An additional 900 to 1000 ml of water is instilled and the descending, transverse, and the ascending colon are examined with the patient in supine position; finally, the cecum is examined with the patient in a slight oblique position.[94]

Limberg reports a 91% sensitivity and 100% specificity for polyps larger than 0.7 cm in diameter; the corresponding values for cancer being 94% and 100%, respectively.[93] This pilot report is rather exciting and several issues need to be addressed in the course of further development and use of the technology.[94]

D. METHANE

Methane (CH_4) is the end product of fermentation by methanogenic bacteria in the intestinal lumen and can rapidly appear in the breath. Patients with cancer of the large intestine have been reported to have high breath methane level (>1 ppm or 0.05 μmol/l), and this assay has been advocated for the screening of patients with colorectal cancer.[95,96] However, subsequent studies have failed to establish its utility as a valid screening test.[97-99]

VII. THE GOLD STANDARD IN DIAGNOSIS

It may come as a surprise to some members of both radiology and endoscopy that the only gold standard there is in the diagnosis to date is histopathological identification of the true nature of the disease that is presumed to have been detected by the initial screening and/or diagnostic assays. One should not be too surprised, as for medical and legal purposes, it is still the standard practice throughout the world for all other diseases, and colon cancer is no exception.

Although as a pathologist I am tempted to give you all the details of the diagnostic criteria, I however feel that such extensive coverage may not be necessary; after all, it is not the intention of this book to make a pathologist out of you in this chapter! The pathology of the precancer and cancer has been discussed in Chapter 2 and the markers for their additional confirmation (precancer) and differential diagnosis in Chapter 3. Suffice it to say that neither the good radiologist or the expert endoscopist could guarantee the diagnosis of an abnormality in many a cases; they certainly identify the lesion and, based on their experience, they can tell us as to their impression. However, more often than not, particularly in cases of small polypoid lesion, the exact diagnosis is often a guess. The suspected lesion is to be biopsied and the specimen must be examined by a trained pathologist.

As in other specialties, the diagnostic ability and accuracy of the specimen is subjected to some inter-pathologist variation. The extent of sampling which, in turn, also depends on the training, experience, continuing education, and motivation of the examining pathologist would also determine the accuracy of the diagnosis. However, a serious limiting factor is the economy. For example, in cases of small lesions, it is important to sample as much of the lesion as possible to determine foci of invasive cancer in an otherwise benign polyp. As discussed in Chapter 2, extension of malignant cells beyond the confinement of *muscularis mucosa* represents a serious lesion and is considered as cancer, while that which has not invaded does not present as bad a prognosis. It may not necessarily be as simple as it sounds; there are situations where the invasion may only be an apparent one and it is important to make the distinction between pseudocarcinomatous invasion and the real one.[100] Then there are issues of the degree of dysplasia, extent of invasion etc., all determining the prognosis. You can gather from the preceding that the more you examine, the more expensive it becomes, with the payoff being better accuracy.

REFERENCES

1. **Fink, D. J.,** Facts about colorectal cancer detection, *Ca.,* 33, 366, 1983.
2. **VanDeen, J.,** Tincture guajaci, und ein Ozontragu, als Reagens auf sehr geringe Blutmengen, namentlich in medico-forensischen Falen, *Arch. Holland Beitr. Natura Heilk,* 3, 228, 1864.
3. **Boas, I.,** Uber okkulte Magenblutungen, *Dtsch. Med. Wochenschr.,* 27, 315, 1901.
4. **Greegor, D. H.,** Diagnosis of large bowel cancer in the asymptomatic colon cancer, *JAMA,* 201, 943, 1967.
5. **Greegor, D. H.,** Occult blood testing for detection of asymptomatic colon cancer, *Cancer,* 28, 131, 1971.
6. **Ransohoff, D. F. and Lang, C. A.,** Small adenomas detected during fecal occult blood test screening for colorectal cancer. The impact of serendipity, *JAMA,* 264, 76, 1990.
7. **Gnauck, R., Macrae, F. A., and Fleisher, M.,** How to perform the fecal occult blood test, *Ca.,* 34, 134, 1984.
8. **Saito, H., Tsuchida, S., Kakizaki, R., Fukushi, M., Sano, M., Aizawa, C., Munakata, A., and Yoshida, Y.,** An immunological occult blood test for mass screening of colorectal cancer by reverse passive hemagglutination (RPHA), *Jap. J. Gastroenterol.,* 81, 2831, 1984.
9. **Hakkinen, I., Paasivuo, R., and Partanen, P.,** Screening of colorectal tumours using an improved faecal occult blood test. Quantitative aspects, *Gut,* 29, 1194, 1988.
10. **Turunen, M. J., Liewendahl, K., Partanen, P., and Adlercreutz, H.,** Immunological detection of faecal occult blood in colorectal cancer, *Br. J. Cancer,* 49, 141, 1984.
11. **Ahlquist, D. A.,** Fecal blood testing: demystifying the occult, in *Gastrointestinal Cancer, Current Approaches to Diagnosis and Treatment,* Levin, B., Ed., University of Texas Press, Austin, TX, 1988, 31.
12. **Ahlquist, D. A., McGill, D. B., Fleming, J. L., Schwartz, S., Wieand, H. S., Rubin, J., and Moertel, C. G.,** Patterns of occult bleeding in asymptomatic colorectal cancer, *Cancer,* 63, 1826, 1989.

13. **Ahlquist, D. A., Klee, G. G., McGill, D. B., and Ellefson, R. D.,** Colorectal cancer detection in practice setting. Impact of fecal blood testing, *Arch. Intern. Med.,* 150, 1041, 1990.
14. **Sampliner, R. E.,** Limitations of fecal occult blood testing, *Arch. Intern. Med.,* 150, 945, 1990.
15. **Lieberman, D. A.,** Colon cancer screening. The dilemma of positive screening tests, *Arch. Intern. Med.,* 150, 740, 1990.
16. **Letsou, G., Ballantyne, G. H., Zdon, M. J., Zucker, K. A., and Modlin, I. M.,** Screening for colorectal neoplasms. A comparison of fecal occult blood test and endoscopic examination, *Dis. Col. Rect.,* 30, 839, 1987.
17. **Stelling H. P., Maimon, H. N., Smith, R. A., Haddy, R. I., and Markert, R. J.,** A comparative study of fecal occult blood tests for early detection of gastrointestinal pathology, *Arch. Intern. Med.,* 150, 1001, 1990.
18. **Johnson, D. A., Gurney, M. S., Volpe, R., Jones, D. M., Van Ness, M. M., Chobanian, S. J., Alvarez, J., Buck, J., Kooyman, G., and Cattau, E. L.,** A prospective study of the prevalence of colonic neoplasms in asymptomatic patients with an age-related risk, *Gastroenterology,* 95, A209, 1988.
19. **Shulman, L., Bernwick, D. M., Caufield, E. A., and Knapp, M. L.,** Detection of colorectal cancer, *Am. Fam. Phys.,* 33, 177, 1986.
20. **Winchester, D. P., Sylvester, J., and Maher, M. L.,** Risks and benefits of mass screening for colorectal neoplasia with the stool guaiac test, *Ca.,* 33, 333, 1983.
21. **Tada, M., Ohtsuka, H., Iso, A., Shimizu, S., Okamura, M., Aoki, Y., and Kawai, K.,** Screening of colorectal cancer by testing rectal mucus for B-D-Gal(1→3)-D-GalNAc (T-antigen), *J. Kyoto Prefect. U. Med.,* 99, 681, 1990.
22. **Seidman, H., Mushinski, M., Gelb, S., and Silverberg, E. S.,** Probabilities of eventually developing or dying of cancer — United States, 1985, *Ca.,* 35, 36, 1985.
23. **Gold, P. and Freedman, S. O.,** Demonstration of tumor-specific antigens in human colonic carcinomata by immunological tolerance and absorption technique, *J. Exp. Med.,* 121, 439, 1965.
24. **Wagener, C., Muller-Wallraf, R., Nisson, S., Groner, J., and Breuer, H.,** Localization and concentration of carcinoembryonic antigen (CEA) in gastrointestinal tumors: correlation with CEA levels in plasma, *J. Natl. Cancer Inst.,* 67, 539, 1981.
25. **Go, V. L., Spencer, R. J., Ravry, M. J., Shorter, R. G., and Huizenga, K. A.,** Carcinoembryonic antigen (CEA) in malignant and inflammatory colonic tissue, *Gastroenterology,* 64,734, 1973.
26. **Thomson, D. M. P., Krupey, J., Freedman, S. O., and Gold., P.,** The radioimmunoassay of circulating carcinoembryonic antigen of the human digestive system, *Proc. Natl. Acad. Sci. U.S.A.,* 64, 161, 1969.
27. **Berson, S. A. and Yalow, R. S.,** Kinetics of reaction between insulin and insulin binding antibody, *J. Clin. Invest.,* 36, 873, 1957.
28. **Yalow, R. S.,** Radioimmunoassay: a probe for the fine structure of biologic systems, *Science,* 200, 1236, 1978.
29. **Engvall, E. and Perlmann, P.,** Enzyme-linked immunosorbent assay, ELISA. III. Quantitation of specific antibodies by enzyme labelled anti-immunoglobulin in antigen-coated tubes, *J. Immunol.,* 109, 129, 1972.
30. **Zamcheck, N. and Kupchick, H. Z.,** Summary of clinical use and limitations of the carcinoembryonic antigen assay and some methodological considerations, in *Manual of Clinical Immunology,* 2nd ed., Rose, N. R. and Friedman, H., Eds., American Society of Microbiology, Washington D.C., 1980, 919.
31. **Welch, J. P.,** Uses of carcinoembryonic antigen determinations in patients with colorectal cancer, in *Colorectal Tumors,* Beahrs, O. H., Higgins, G. A., and Weinstein, J. J., Eds., J. B. Lippincott, Philadelphia, 1986, 139.
32. **Kievit, J. and van de Velde, C. J. H.,** Utility and cost of carcinoembryonic antigen monitoring in colon cancer follow-up evaluation, a Markov analysis, *Cancer,* 65, 2580, 1990.
33. **Hoff, H. C.,** Retrograde intubation of the cecum, *AJR,* 20, 226, 1928.
34. **Baird, J. L.,** British Patent No. 20,969/27, 1927.
35. **Lamm, H.,** Flexible optical instruments, *Z. Instr.,* 50, 579, 1930.
36. **Hopkins, H. H. and Kapany, N. S.,** A flexible fibrescope using static scanning, *Nature (London),* 173, 39, 1954.
37. **Van Heel, A. C. S.,** A new method of transporting optical images without aberrations, *Nature (London),* 173, 39, 1954.
38. **Hirschowitz, B. I., Peters, C. W., and Curtis, L. E.,** Preliminary report on a long fiberscope for examination of stomach and duodenum, *Univ. Mich. Med. Bull.,* 23, 178, 1957.
39. **Matsunaga, F., Tsushima, H., and Kuboto, T.,** Photography of the colon, *Gastroenterol. Endosc. (Tokyo),* 1, 58, 1959.
40. **Niwa, H.,** On photography of colon and pharynx using gastrocamera, *Gastroenterol. Endosc. (Tokyo),* 2, 77, 1960.
41. **Niwa, H., Utsumi, Y., Kaneko, E., Nakamura, T., Fujino, M., Kasumi, A., Yoshida, A., Matsumoto, M., Yoshitoshi, Y.,** Clinical experience of colonic fiberscope, *Gastroenterol. Endosc. (Tokyo),* 11, 163, 1969.
42. **Overholt, B. F.,** Flexible fiberoptic sigmoidoscope, *Ca.,* 19, 81, 1969.
43. **Wolff, W. I.,** Colonoscopy: history and development, *Am. J. Gastroenterol.,* 84, 1017, 1989.
44. **Wolff, W. I. and Shinya, H.,** Colonofiberoscopy: diagnostic modality and therapeutic application, *Bull. Soc. Int. Chir.,* 5, 525, 1971.

45. **Sugarbaker, P. H.,** Fiberoptic colonoscopy, in *Colorectal tumors,* Beahrs, O. H., Higgins, G. A., and Weinstein, J. J., Eds., Lippincott, Philadelphia, 1986, 123.

46. **Brenna, E., Skreden, K., Waldum, H. L., Marvik, R., Dybdahl, J. H., Kleveland, P. M., Sandvik, A. K., Halvorsen, T., Myrvold, H. E., and Petersen, H.,** The benefit of colonoscopy, *Scand. J. Gastroenterol.,* 25, 81, 1990.

47. **Kolata, G.,** Debate over colon cancer screening, *Science,* 229, 636, 1985.

48. **McGill, D. B.,** The president and the power of colonoscope, *Mayo Clin. Proc.,* 60, 886, 1985.

49. **Neugut, A. I. and Forde, K. A.,** Screening colonoscopy: has the time come?, *Am. J. Gastroenterol.,* 83, 295, 1988.

50. **Ferrands, P. A., Vellacott, K. D., Amar, S. S., Balfour, T. W., and Hardcastle, J. W.,** Flexible fiberoptic sigmoidoscopy and double-contrast barium-enema examination in the identification of adenomas and carcinoma of the colon, *Dis. Colon Rectum,* 26, 727, 1983.

51. **Cancer Economics,** Radiologists call barium enema most cost effective colon screen, *Cancer Lett.,* 15, 1 (Suppl.), 1989.

52. **Olmsted, W. W.,** Barium enema in the early diagnosis of colonic malignancy, in *Colorectal tumors,* Beahrs, O. H., Higgins, G. A., and Weinstein, J. J., Eds., Lippincott, Philadelphia, 1986, 49.

53. **Lipkin, M., Friedman, E., Winawer, S. J., and Newmark, H.,** Colonic epithelial cell proliferation in responders and nonresponders to supplementary dietary calcium, *Cancer Res.,* 49, 248, 1989.

54. **Deschner, E. E.,** Kinetics of normal, preneoplastic, and neoplastic colonic epithelium, in *Colon Cancer Cells,* Moyer, M. P. and Poste, G. H., Eds., Academic Press, San Diego, CA, 1990, 41.

55. **Cole, J. W. and McKalen, A.,** Observations of cell renewals in normal rectal mucosa *in vivo* with thymidine-H[3], *Gastroenterology,* 41, 122, 1961.

56. **Deschner, E. E., Lewis, C. M., and Lipkin, M.,** *In vitro* study of human epithelial cells. I. Atypical zone of ^{3}H-thymidine incorporation in mucosa of multiple polyposis, *J. Clin. Invest.,* 42, 1922, 1963.

57. **Deschner, E. E., Lipkin, M., and Solomon, C.,** *In vitro* study of human epithelial cells. II. ^{3}H-Thymidine incorporation into polyps and adjacent mucosa, *J. Natl. Cancer Inst.,* 36, 849, 1966.

58. **Deschner, E. E. and Lipkin, M.,** Proliferative patterns in colonic mucosa in familial polyposis, *Cancer,* 35, 413, 1975.

59. **Maskens, A. P. and Deschner, E.E.,** Tritiated thymidine incorporation into epithelial cells of normal-appearing colorectal mucosa of cancer patients, *J. Natl. Cancer Inst.,* 58, 1221, 1977.

60. **Deschner, E. E. and Maskens, A. P.,** Significance of the labeling index and labeling distribution as kinetic parameters in colorectal mucosa of cancer patients and DMH treated animals, *Cancer,* 50, 1136, 1982.

61. **James, J. T., Shamsuddin, A. M., and Trump, B. F.,** Comparative study of the morphological, histochemical, and proliferative changes induced in the large intestine if ICR/Ha and C57Bl/Ha mice by 1,2-dimethylhydrazine, *J. Natl. Cancer Inst.,* 71, 955, 1983.

62. **Richards, T. C.,** Changes in crypt cell populations of mouse colon during recovery from treatment with 1,2-dimethylhydrazine, *J. Natl. Cancer Inst.,* 66, 907, 1981.

63. **Tutton, P. J. and Barkla, D. H.,** Cell proliferation in the descending colon of dimethylhydrazine-treated rats and in dimethylhydrazine-induced adenocarcinoma, *Virchows Arch. (Cell Pathol.),* 24, 147, 1976.

64. **Gratzner, H. G.,** Monoclonal antibody to 5-bromo- and 5-iododeoxyuridine: a new reagent for detection of DNA replication, *Science,* 218, 474, 1982.

65. **Cawood, A. H. and Savage, J. R. K.,** A comparison of the use of bromodeoxyuridine and [^{3}H]thymidine in studies of the cell cycle, *Cell Tissue Kinet.,* 16, 51, 1983.

66. **Morstyn, G., Hsu, S. M., Kinsella, T., Gratzner, H., Russo, A., and Mitchell, J. B.,** Bromodeoxyuridine in tumors and chromosomes detected with a monoclonal antibody, *J. Clin. Invest.,* 72, 1844, 1983.

67. **Morstyn, G., Pyke, K., Gardner, J., Ashcroft, R., de Fazio, A., and Bhathal, P.,** Immunohistochemical identification of proliferating cells in organ culture using bromodeoxyuridine and a monoclonal antibody, *J. Histochem. Cytochem.,* 34, 697, 1986.

68. **Welberg, J. W. M., De Vries, E. G. E., Hardonk, M. J., Mulder, N. H., Harms, G., Grond, J., Zwart, N., Koudstaal, J., De Ley, L., and Kleibeuker, J. H.,** Proliferation rate of colonic mucosa in normal subjects and patients with colonic neoplasms: a refined immunohistochemical method, *J. Clin. Pathol.,* 43, 453, 1990.

69. **Bleiberg, H., Buyse, M., and Galand, P.,** Cell kinetic indicators of premalignant stages of colorectal cancer, *Cancer,* 56,124, 1985.

70. **Terpstra, O. T., van Blankenstein, M., Dees, J., and Eilers, G. A. M.,** Abnormal pattern of cell proliferation in the entire colonic mucosa of patients with colon adenoma or cancer, *Gastroenterology,* 92, 704, 1987.

71. **Shamsuddin, A. K. M. and Trump, B. F.,** Colon epithelium. I. Light microscopic, histochemical and ultrastructural features of normal colon epithelium of male Fischer-344 rats, *J. Natl. Cancer Inst.,* 66, 375, 1981.

72. **Shamsuddin, A. M., Phelps, P. C., and Trump, B. F.,** Human large intestinal epithelium: light microscopy, histochemistry and ultrastructure, *Human Pathol.,* 13, 790, 1982.

73. **James, J. T., Shamsuddin, A. M., and Trump, B. F.,** A comparative study of the normal histochemical and proliferative properties of the large intestine in ICR/Ha and C57Bl/Ha mice, *Virchows Arch. (Cell Pathol.)* 41, 133, 1982.

74. **Sunter, J. P., Watson, A. J., Wright, N. A., and Appleton, D. R.,** Cell proliferation at different sites along the length of the rat colon, *Virchows Arch. (Cell Pathol.),* 32, 753, 1979.

75. **Appleton, D. R., Sunter, J. P., deRodriguez, M. S. B., and Watson, A. J.,** Cell proliferation in the mouse large bowel, with details of the analyses of the experimental data, in *Cell Proliferation in the Gastrointestinal Tract,* Appleton, D. R., Sunter, J. P., and Watson, A. J., Eds., Pitman Medical, Tunbridge, Kent, England, 1980, 40.

76. **Roncucci, L., Ponz de Leon, M., Scalmati, A., Malagoli, G., Pratissoli, S., Perini, M., and Chahin, N. J.,** The influence of age on colonic epithelial cell proliferation, *Cancer,* 62, 2373, 1988.

77. **Chang, W. W. L.,** Renewal of the epithelium in the descending colon of mouse. II. Diurnal variation in the proliferative activity of epithelial cells, *Am. J. Anat.,* 131, 111, 1971.

78. **Hamilton, E.,** Diurnal variation in proliferative compartments and their relation to cryptogenic cells in the mouse colon, *Cell Tissue Kinet.,* 12, 91, 1979.

79. **Shamsuddin, A. K. M., Barrett, L. A., Autrup, H., Harris, C. C., and Trump, B. F.,** Long-term organ culture of adult rat colon, *Pathol. Res. Pract.,* 163, 362, 1978.

80. **Shamsuddin, A. K. M.,** Colon organ culture as a model for carcinogenesis, in *Colon Cancer Cells,* Moyer, M. P. and Poste, G. H., Eds., Academic Press, San Diego, CA, 1990, 137.

81. **O'Brien, T. G., Simsiman, R. C., and Boutwell, R. K.,** Induction of the polyamine-biosynthetic enzymes in mouse epidermis by tumor promoting agents, *Cancer Res.,* 35, 1662, 1975.

82. **Luk, G. D. and Baylin, S. B.,** Ornithine decarboxylase as a biologic marker in familial colonic polyposis, *N. Engl. J. Med.,* 311, 80, 1984.

83. **LaMuraglia, G. M., Lacaine, F., and Malt, R. A.,** High ornithine decarboxylase activity and polyamine levels in human colorectal neoplasia, *Ann. Surg.,* 204, 89, 1986.

84. **Loser, C., Folsch, U. R., Paprotny, C., and Creutzfeldt, W.,** Polyamines in colorectal cancer. Evaluation of polyamine concentrations in colon tissue, serum, and urine of 50 patients with colorectal cancer, *Cancer,* 65, 958, 1990.

85. **Giardiello, F. M., Theiss, H. W., and Luk, G. D.,** Human colon adenocarcinoma cell growth is inhibited by a combination of *cis*-diamminedichloroplatinum and difluoromethulornithine, *Gastroenterology,* 88, 1392, 1985.

86. **Luk, G. D., Desai, T. K., Bull, A. W., Kinzie, J. L., Thompson, R. R., Silverman, A. L., and Moshier, J.,** Rectal mucosal ornithine decarboxylase activity as a marker for colonic polyps and cancer, *Gastroenterology,* 94, A272, 1988.

87. **Mamont, P. S., Duchesne, M.-C., Grove, J., and Bey, P.,** Antiproliferative properties of DL-α-difluoromethyl-ornithine in cultured cells. A consequence of the irreversible inhibition of ODC, *Biochem. Biophys. Res. Commun.,* 81, 58, 1978.

88. **Seiler, N., Danzin, C., Prakash, N. J., and Koch-Weser, J.,** Effects of ornithine decarboxylase inhibitors *in vivo,* in *Enzyme-Activated Irreversible Inhibitors,* Seiler, N., Jung, M. J., and Koch-Weser, J., Eds., Elsevier, New York, 1978, 55.

89. **Marton, L. J., Levin, V. A., Hervatin, S. J., Koch-Weser, J., McCann, P. P., and Sjoerdsma, A.,** Potentiation of the antitumor therapeutic effects of 1,3-bis(2-chloroethyl)-1-nitrosourea by α-difluoromethylornithine, an ornithine decarboxylase inhibitor, *Cancer Res.,* 41, 4436, 1981.

90. **Luk, G. D., Abeloff, M. D., Griffin, C. A., and Baylin, S. B.,** Successful treatment with DL-α-difluoromethylornithine in established human small cell variant lung carcinoma implants in athymic nude mice, *Cancer Res.,* 43, 4239, 1983.

91. **Tempero, M. A., Nishioka, K., Knott, K., and Zetterman, R. K.,** Chemoprevention of mouse colon tumors with difluoromethylornithine during and after carcinogen treatment, *Cancer Res.,* 49, 5793, 1989.

92. **Robertson, F. M., Gilmour, S. K., Conney, A. H., Huang, M.-T., Beavis, A. J., Laskin, J. D., Hietala, O. A., and O'Brien, T. G.,** Identification of epidermal cell subpopulations with increased ornithine decarboxylase activity following treatment of mouse epidermis with 12-*O*-tetradecanoylphorbol-13-acetate, *Cancer Res.,* 50, 4741, 1990.

93. **Limberg, B.,** Diagnosis of large bowel tumours by colonic sonography, *Lancet,* 335, 144, 1990.

94. **Limberg, B.,** Colonic sonography, (reply to letter), *Lancet,* 335, 144, 1990.

95. **Haines, A., Metz, G., Dilawari, J., Blendis, L. M., and Wiggins, M.,** Breath methane in patients with cancer of the large bowel, *Lancet,* 2, 481, 1977.

96. **Pique, J. M., Pallares, M., Cuso, E., Vilar Bonet, J., and Gassahall, M. A.,** Methane production and colon cancer, *Gastroenterology,* 87,601, 1984.

97. **Karlin, D. A., Jones, R. D., Stroehlein, J. R., Mastromarino, A. J., and Potter, G. D.,** Breath methane excretion in patients with unresected colon cancer, *J. Natl. Cancer Inst.,* 69, 573, 1982.

98. **McKay, L. F., Eastwood, M. A., and Brydon, W. G.,** Methane excretion in man — a study of breath, flatus and feces, *Gut,* 26, 69, 1985.

99. **Kashtan, H., Rabau, M., Peled, Y., Milstein, A., and Wiznitzer, Th.,** Methane production in patients with colorectal carcinoma, *Isr. J. Med. Sci.,* 25, 614, 1989.

100. **Fenoglio-Preiser, C. M. and Pascal, R. R.,** Other tumors of the large intestine. I. Epithelial tumors, in *Gastrointestinal and Oesophageal Pathology,* Whitehead, R., Ed., Churchill Livingstone, New York, 1989, 747.

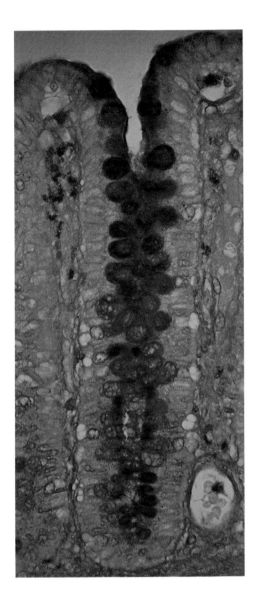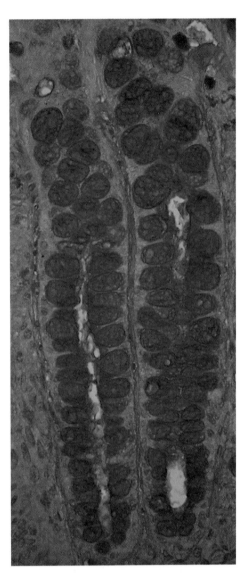

PLATE 1. A crypt from the ascending colon of a normal individual, showing predominantly magenta colored neutral mucin and slight mixed neutral and acidic mucin (purple) by alcian blue-PAS sequence (left). Rectal crypts from the same individual, identically stained with alcian blue-PAS sequence show almost exclusive presence of acidic mucin in the mucous cells (right). (From Shamsuddin, A. M., Phelps, P. C., and Trump, B. F., *Hum. Pathol.*, 13, 790, 1982. With permission.)

INTERPRETING THE HEMOCCULT® BRAND TEST

Negative Smears

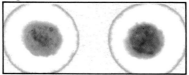

Sample report: negative
No detectable blue on or at the edge of the smears indicates the test is negative for occult blood. (See **LIMITATIONS OF PROCEDURE**.)

Negative and Positive Smears

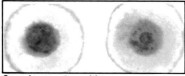

Positive Smears

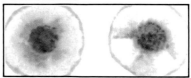

Sample report: positive
Any trace of blue on or at the edge of one or more of the smears indicates the test is positive for occult blood.

PLATE 5. A typical guaiac test for qualitative detection of FOB (Hemoccult®) showing brown color of fecal material and blue coloration of FOB positive samples. Courtesy of William F. Ulrich, Ph.D., SmithKline Diagnostics, San Jose, CA.

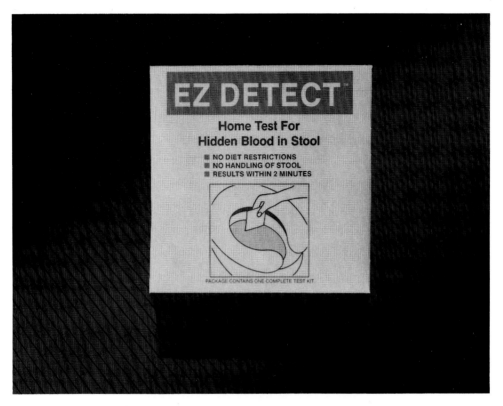

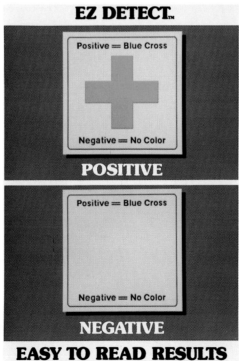

PLATE 6. EZ Detect™, a nonguaiac test for qualitative detection of FOB in the toilet bowl (above); this kit appears to be aesthetically more acceptable and may enhance patient compliance. A typical positive (blue) color reaction indicating the presence of blood (below). Note the similarity of final blue color reaction with the guaiac tests. Courtesy of Mr. Zackary S. Irani, Biomerica Inc., Newport Beach, CA.

Illustrated Test Procedure

Standard Test

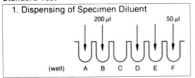
1. Dispensing of Specimen Diluent

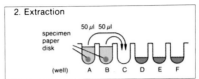
2. Extraction

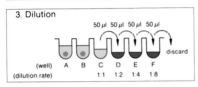
3. Dilution

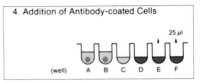
4. Addition of Antibody-coated Cells

Positive Control

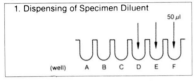
1. Dispensing of Specimen Diluent

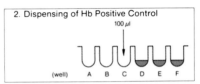
2. Dispensing of Hb Positive Control

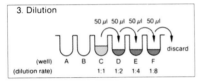
3. Dilution

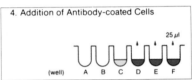
4. Addition of Antibody-coated Cells

Negative Control

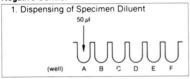
1. Dispensing of Specimen Diluent

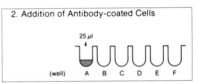
2. Addition of Antibody-coated Cells

For convenient reference, remove and post near work area.

PLATE 7. Schematic diagram of the steps involved in the immunological FOBT (HemeSe-lect™). Courtesy of William F. Ulrich, Ph.D., SmithKline Diagnostics, San Jose, CA.

Interpreting the HemeSelect™ Test

Specimen Extract

Specimen Disk | Specimen Extract Dilutions

Sample Result

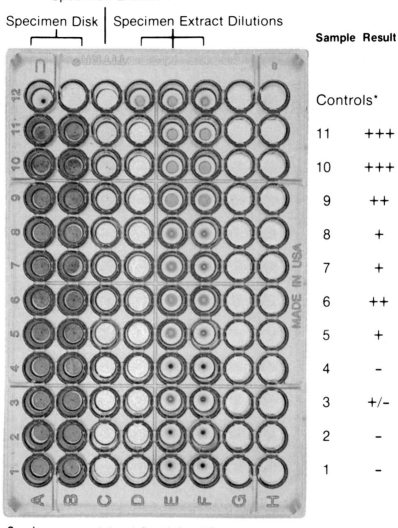

Sample	Result
Controls*	
11	+++
10	+++
9	++
8	+
7	+
6	++
5	+
4	-
3	+/-
2	-
1	-

Specimen Dilution   1:1   1:2   1:4   1:8

* In the control row, the negative control in well A displays a negative reaction and the positive control in wells D, E, and F shows various positive patterns in proportion to the concentration of Hb positive control they contain.

PLATE 8. A 96-well microtiter plate showing positive and negative reverse passive hemagglutination obtained by HemeSelect™. Courtesy of William F. Ulrich, Ph.D., SmithKline Diagnostics, San Jose, CA.

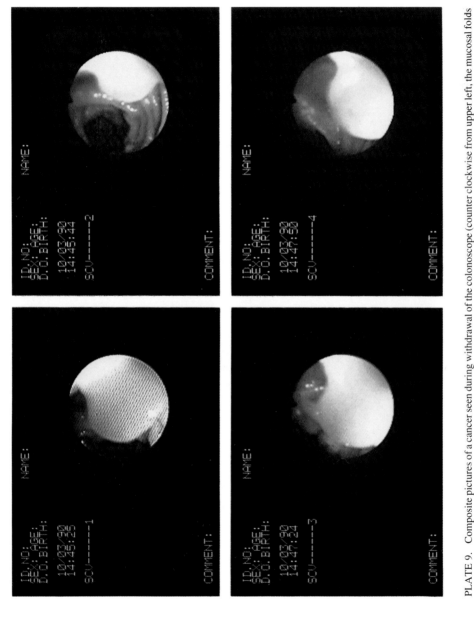

PLATE 9. Composite pictures of a cancer seen during withdrawal of the colonoscope (counter clockwise from upper left, the mucosal folds can be seen in the upper right). Courtesy of Jahangir M. Khan, M.D., and Daliah K. Shamsuddin, M.D. Franklin Square Hospital, Baltimore, MD.

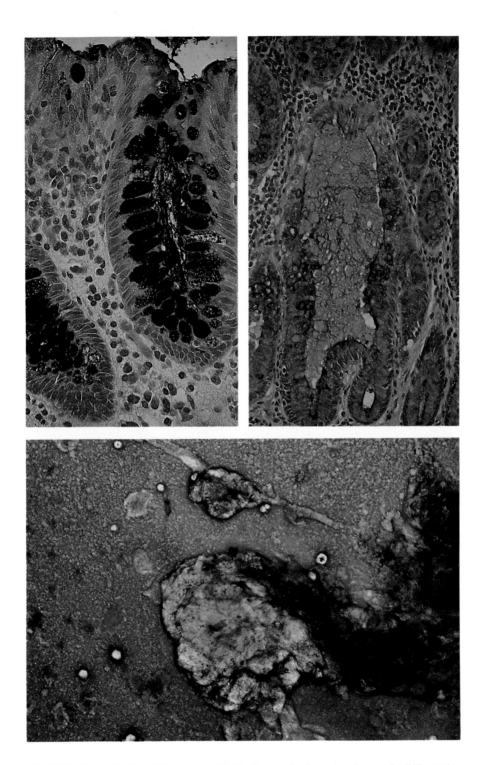

PLATE 10. The origination of the concept of field effect mucin change in colon and feasibility testing with sialomucin. The upper left picture is that of a colonic crypt from a normal individual without known cancer or precancer of the colon showing normal test tube shape and normally occurring brown-black sulfomucin. The crypt in the upper right is remote from a cancer, showing distorted crypt with abnormal blue sialomucin seen also in known cancer and precancer. The bottom figure is the rectal mucus taken from a patient with carcinoma of the cecum, smeared on the glass slide, and high iron diamine-alcian blue (HID-AB) staining was performed. Note the blue colored sialomucin amongst normal sulfomucin.

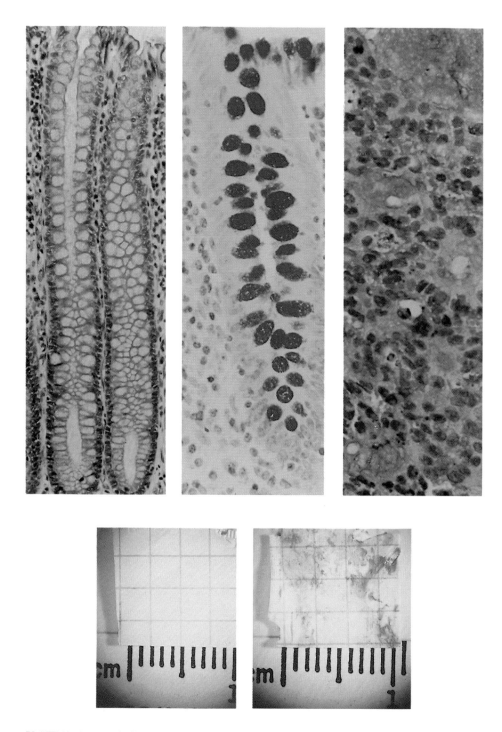

PLATE 11. A composite illustration of both tissue and rectal mucus galactose oxidase reaction. The upper left is a normal human colon showing regular test tube shaped glands with no reactivity with galactose oxidase-Schiff's sequence. A histological section of a colonic adenocarcinoma showing galactose oxidase positive reaction is at the upper right. The upper middle picture is that of a morphologically normal crypt, remote from a cancer, showing strong reactivity to galactose oxidase-Schiff. The galactose oxidase reaction in the rectal mucus of a normal (negative) and a cancer patient (positive with magenta coloration) is shown in the lower left and right panels, respectively.

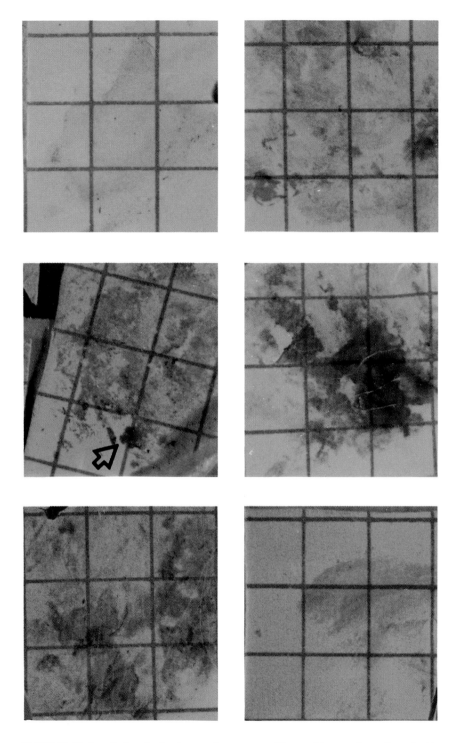

PLATE 12. Various shades of color that may be encountered in a positive sample are shown in this illustration. All the samples except the bottom right are positive. Note that the top left is light pink and areas of magenta can be appreciated within the brown perhaps fecal pigmentation (arrow) in the middle left filter. Note that a magenta coloration, however small, is a positive reaction. The commercially available kits are expected to have color charts and other quality control measures for consistency and better accuracy.

Chapter 5

NEW ASSAYS FOR DETECTION OF COLON CANCER AND PRECANCER

I. INTRODUCTION

As discussed in Chapter 3, the alteration in mucin biochemistry of both the intracellular and the secreted mucus in the large intestine is a consistent marker that emerges during the formation of cancer of the large intestine and has been validated both in the experimental models and in humans.[1-4] Consistent with its emergence during cancer formation is its expression in various conditions of the large intestine that are known to carry a high risk of subsequent progression to cancer (e.g., polyps, inflammatory bowel diseases, etc.). The altered mucin is expressed not only in the cells that are cancerous and precancerous, but is also found in the otherwise morphologically normal appearing cells away from the cancer. Observation of mucin abnormalities in the normal-appearing mucosa away from cancer was not new. Filipe and Branfoot[5] had earlier made such observation; its exact significance was however not understood, perhaps in view of the rigid adherence to the "polyp-cancer only" theory of genesis of colon cancer. Based on parallel *in vivo, in vitro* studies in experimental models, extrapolation of the finding, and comparison with human tissues bearing cancer or precancer, I forwarded an explanation for this phenomenon as being the result of generalized field effect of the carcinogenic stimuli.[1,4] I had also proposed that in light of these observed changes, it should be possible to devise alternate strategies for early detection of cancerous events.[1,4]

I soon embarked on the feasibility of detecting the abnormal mucus in the rectum of patients with cancer of the large intestine. Glen Jockle, a resident physician in Pathology, expressed interest in working with me. E. George Elias, Professor of the Department of Surgery at the University of Maryland, had provided the rectal mucus samples which were smeared on microscopic glass slides from patients; Glen and I analyzed for the presence of the abnormal sialomucin (Plate 10, see color plates*). Initially, we had rather exciting results; several of the patients who had cancer of the colon and even cecum scored positive. However, the technical difficulty, the long reaction time (nearly 2 d) and, later, some unexpected results led me to consider an alternate and more definitive marker.

In 1982, Boland at al.[6] and Cooper[7] presented evidence that the T antigen (see Chapter 3) is expressed in the cancer of colon and not in the normal human large intestinal mucosa. Glen and I investigated the expression of the marker in our animal model by using peanut lectin, needless to say that we were excited to find its differential expression in the morphologically normal-appearing mucosa of animals treated with colon carcinogen, and dysplastic and carcinomatous foci, but not in normal untreated control animals. Alaaeldeen M. Elsayed from Egypt joined my laboratory as a graduate student and I had him validate our observation in the human precancer as well as cancer.[8] I then embarked on exploiting the property of peanut agglutinin to competitively bind to neuraminidase-treated human red blood cells and the rectal mucus of patients with colonic cancer and precancer, both of which appear to have the same sugar residue D-Gal-$\beta(1\rightarrow3)$-D-GalNAc. Soon after Glen and I had developed the hemagglutination inhibition assay, Glen finished his training in pathology and left for private practice, a rather wise decision at a time when research funds were (and still are) rapidly diminishing. With the rectal mucus samples of patients provided by my wife Daliah, an internist, and a gastroenterologist friend Jahangir Khan, we then performed a pilot clinical study on the

---

* See color plates following page 102.

hemagglutination inhibition assay.[9] Although the result of hemagglutination inhibition assay was encouraging, the quest for a simpler test was still on.

Around this time, Schulte and Spicer[10] reported the technique of galactose oxidase-Schiff sequence to identify D-Gal-β(1$\rightarrow$3)-D-GalNAc residues in rodent tracheal tissue sections. We thus embarked on its application in the tissue sections of precancer and cancer of the large intestine.[11] Having demonstrated the usefulness of the galactose oxidase-Schiff sequence in the tissue, I then explored the feasibility of the technique in identifying D-Gal-β(1$\rightarrow$3)-D-GalNAc in the rectal mucus. The first problem was to find a suitable substrate for immobilizing the mucus glycoprotein which was rather easily resolved by using nitrocellulose filters. However, subsequent experiments resulted in a uniform magenta coloration of the entire filter. These problems were frustrating to the point that Elsayed declared "it wouldn't work" and wished not to pursue the issue any more. With a little help from scientific knowledge, common sense, and perseverance, I finally identified the proper protein-capturing membrane filter and the proper sequence of reactions in obtaining the magenta color for the abnormal mucus. Also, the normal mucus was unreactive, showing little background noise. Using patients from hospitals and doctors' offices, once again provided by my wife Daliah and our friend Jahangir Khan, the test then underwent pilot clinical study. All 13 patients with cancer scored positive and so were only 4 of 58 asymptomatic subjects.

You can imagine that we were excited and wanted to let others know. We were in luck; there was still time to submit an abstract to the 76th Annual Meeting of the U.S.-Canadian division of the International Academy of Pathology, now called U.S.-Canadian Academy of Pathology (USCAP) to convene in Chicago in March, 1987. Either the USCAP was badly in need of publicity or the organizers, particularly Nathan Kaufman, continued to like me, or both; I was contacted for writing a "lay" summary for the press. Needless to say, Elsayed and I became famous (perhaps only to our families and close friends!). You all know that fame in medicine comes only from having your paper published in *The New England Journal of Medicine,* and I thought, "why not?" But alas, that elusive fame did not come; our material was not earth shaking, I guess! Meanwhile, at the USCAP meeting in Chicago, Bernard Wagner, then Editor of *Human Pathology,* asked me to send him the manuscript; he even hinted that following the usual peer review, he would expedite the publication. Since we failed to become famous by publishing the paper in *The New England Journal of Medicine,* or even *JAMA* and *The Lancet,* I thought it time to take Barney up on his offer. Wagner, a perfect gentleman, did not renege on his offer of expediting the publication and the paper saw the light of day.[12] Note that we refrained from using a catchy title; by now, if you have gone through the rigorous criteria set forth by WHO for screening tests (Chapter 1), you would know why. Certainly, we discussed that possibility, but did not want to prematurely claim it in the title.

Inasmuch as the galactose oxidase test appeared to be a very simple yet accurate assay, it nonetheless is qualitative. Since the marker sugar moiety is expressed in different precancerous conditions of variable risk for malignancy, it seemed like a good idea to come up with a quantitative assay which could determine the amount of marker per unit of mucous glycoprotein. My experience in enzyme immunoassays, such as BALIA (biotin-avidin-linked immunoassay)[13] and USERIA (ultrasensitive enzyme linked radioimmunoassay),[14] came handy and soon enough I had developed a avidin-biotin lectin enzyme immunoassay.[15] Inspired by Glen's suggestion for a quick "pregnancy test" type assay, I had also developed a latex agglutination assay;[15] Elsayed, by this time had decided not to pursue graduate studies and research in my laboratory and left for better opportunities.

Since the galactose oxidase test has undergone the most extensive investigation, I shall describe it first. The latex agglutination and the avidin-biotin lectin enzyme immunoassay are yet to be evaluated in a clinical setting and, therefore, will be described in Chapter 6.

II. GALACTOSE OXIDASE TEST

A. BACKGROUND AND PRINCIPLE
The following factors are important in understanding the principle of this assay:

1. The carcinogenic stimuli, responsible for the cancer of the colon, are perhaps in the feces or are delivered to the large intestine through blood circulation. In any event, they would induce multiple foci of precancerous and cancerous changes in the entire large intestine (field effect); some of these alterations are recognizable only as biochemical changes of mucin glycoprotein.
2. Therefore, it is likely that the mucus of the rectum, being part of the large intestine, would also share the same abnormalities. Digital rectal examination is also a part of routine physical examination and it is rather automatic that the examining gloved finger will contain some mucus for sampling at no additional inconvenience either to the patient or to the physician.
3. The mucus in patients with cancer or precancerous conditions and lesions reacts with galactose oxidase. Specifically, the enzyme oxidizes the C-6 hydroxyl groups of both galactose and galactosamine subunits [D-Gal-β(1→3)-D-GalNAc] of the mucus glycoprotein to produce aldehyde groups. Subsequently, Schiff's basic fuchsin dye which reacts with vicinal aldehydes render the substance magenta (Figure 1 and Plate 11, see color plates*).
4. The mucus (either in the rectum or elsewhere in the large intestine) in the normal subject does not react with galactose oxidase, and therefore does not yield a magenta coloration on subsequent staining with Schiff's basic fuchsin dye.

B. METHODS
Although the total reaction time of the initial assays were less than 2 h, considerable prior preparation was necessary for successful assay.[12] Subsequent modifications have rendered the assay even more simple with the results obtained in less than 15 min. The following are the steps of procedure:

1. Smear mucus on test strip
2. React with galactose oxidase (10 min at room temperature)
3. Wash with distilled water (optional)
4. React with Schiff's basic fuchsin (1 min)
5. Rinse in running tap water
6. Look for pink/magenta/purple coloration when dry (air-dry, oven, hot plate)

As a part of a routine physical examination, a complete digital rectal examination is to be performed on the individual. Use only a minimal amount of lubricant, since one is collecting mucus which is also slimy in nature. Rotate the examining finger 360° to examine the adjacent organs such as the prostate, uterus, etc. Following completion of the rectal examination, smear the mucus on the labeled side of the membrane and let air-dry. The assay can be done immediately or at a later period. Once the mucus is smeared on the membrane, it is stable for at least a year. An area of magenta coloration, however small or large, is the positive reaction, indicating that the patient may have cancer, precancerous polyp, or other diseases of the colorectum and therefore is a candidate for further evaluation.

What does a negative reaction mean? A negative reaction may mean that either: (a) there is no abnormal mucus in the rectum, or (b) the sampling itself was inadequate, resulting in the

---

* See color plates following page 102.

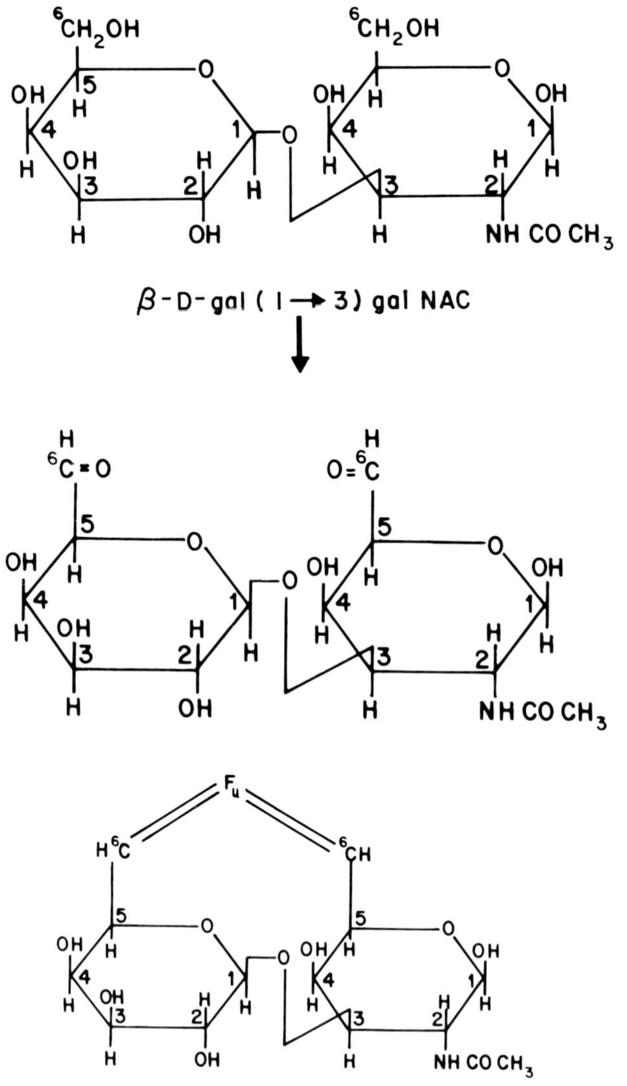

FIGURE 1. Current concept of the mechanism of galactose oxidase-Schiff reaction for detecting D-Gal-β(1→3)-D-GalNAc. Perhaps the absence of a blocking sialic acid in cancerous and precancerous mucous glycoprotein allows galactose oxidase to oxidize the alcohol group at C-6 positions, yielding aldehyde groups. Schiff's basic fuchsin then reacts with the two vicinyl aldehydes to impart magenta coloration.

absence of any mucus, normal or abnormal. This latter phenomenon may give rise to false negative result due to technical error and clearly, a technique or process had to be devised to differentiate between the two. Since periodic acid is known to oxidize the alcohol groups of sugar residues in a nonspecific manner, I had rationalized that a periodic acid-Schiff sequence in galactose oxidase negative samples would be worth trying. This came about the time when I was experiencing some vague lower gastrointestinal symptoms myself, and I decided to assay my own mucus sample. It was galactose oxidase negative, but I wanted to be sure that it was not technically negative and, thus, pilot tested the periodic acid-Schiff sequence.

Perhaps it is needless to say that it worked. Therefore, to ensure that the negative test result is not due to inadequate sampling I recommend the following additional step:

7.   Add 2 drops of periodic acid and react for 5 min; then, repeat steps 3 and 4.

A positive reaction (purple or magenta) indicates that the sampling was adequate, but the patient was negative for the abnormal mucus; in that event, the assay is to be repeated every 6 months.

If one does not obtain a purple or magenta color, it means that the sample does not have any mucus. Please obtain another sample and repeat steps 2 through 6.

Precautions to be taken include:

1.   The sampling membrane should be clean; do not touch the membrane except to smear the mucus sample.
2.   Store reagents in refrigerator at around 4°C.
3.   Avoid spilling Schiff's reagent and use care while rinsing, since the dye may make your clothes more colorful.
4.   Color interpretations can sometimes be tricky. A positive reaction is usually an obvious pink or magenta or even purple; a light pink is found when the intensity of reaction is weak and purple when it is very strong, with magenta being the most common (Plate 12, see color plates*). A magenta or red color, however small, is to be interpreted as positive; our extensive research with tissue galactose oxidase reaction demonstrates that in carcinomas also one may occasionally find only a small focus of positive reaction.

The feces which are washed off during the process do not interfere with the color reaction. Even if there is residual feces, since it is usually brown, it does not pose a great problem in discriminating from the positive pink-magenta-purple. These minor but important issues have been addressed by the commercial manufacturers, and necessary steps have been taken to alleviate them by incorporating color charts in the kits.

C. RESTRICTIONS

To date, I am not aware of any dietary substances that may interfere with the assay. Thus, unlike the fecal occult blood tests (FOBTs), there are no dietary restrictions to be followed for this assay and the reason for this would be evident from a review of the principle of the two assays. Briefly, the FOBTs are based on the principle of detecting hemoglobin or other substances with peroxidase-like activity and many dietary substances are to be abstained from for proper conduction of the FOBTs. On the other hand, the mucin abnormality in the galactose oxidase test is due to carcinogenic alterations of the cellular phenotype. However, a few points need to be clarified.

1.   The sampling and the effect of the lubricant. In the performance of digital rectal examination, it is necessary to use lubricants for minimizing patient discomfort. Therefore, we tested the effect of various lubricants used by the physicians and our experience indicates that the type of lubricant used does not have any effect on the outcome of the test. However, the amount of lubricant may affect the sampling of mucus itself, since too much lubricant (a slimy substance) would interfere with the collection of adequate mucus which is also slimy in nature. Thus, the use of a minimal amount of lubricant without inducing patient discomfort is recommended.
2.   It is not usual to perform a screening test in a colonoscopy clinic since patients who are candidates for colonoscopy are already referred there because of abnormal screening

* See color plates following page 102.

TABLE 1
Galactose Oxidase Test Results (Pilot Study)[12]

Cancer	Neoplastic polyp	High risk/ symptomatic	Asymptomatic "normal"	Total
13/13	1/1	1/1	4/58	73
100%			6.9%	

Note: Numbers are positive test results / total in each category.

TABLE 2
Evaluation of Galactose Oxidase Test in Japan (Sakamoto Study I)[19]

Cancer	Precancer polyp, UC, CD	Negative colonoscopy[a]	Specificity
8/10 (80%)	8/11 (73%)	17/45 (38%)	62%

[a] Patients came to Surgical clinic for anal or rectal diseases, complete colonoscopy not performed in all cases.

test results. In the event that such studies are undertaken, please be advised that colonoscopy "preps" themselves do not interfere with the chemical reaction; however, the dilutional effect on the mucus interferes with sampling and results in smudging and, therefore, interpretation of color reaction.

3. Occasionally, mucus samples are encountered which are watery in nature, often seen in patients with villous adenoma or mucinous carcinomas. This results in the migration of the mucus glycoprotein to the opposite side of the membrane. Thus, it is good practice to examine both sides of the membrane before scoring a sample as negative.

D. SUMMARY OF PERFORMANCE

The data from the pilot study is presented in Table 1, which shows excellent sensitivity and specificity. One of the major criticisms of the pilot study is the lack of documentation of the false negative rate; that is, in the absence of colonoscopic evaluation ("gold standard") of all tested subjects, how could one be certain that the 58 noncancer, nonpolyp individuals did not have any lesion? This issue however poses a serious problem. First, in the current day and age, the cost and discomfort of colonoscopy cannot be justified in asymptomatic individuals. Therefore, one has to rely on patients who are seen in a colonoscopy clinic; the presence or absence of a visible neoplasm can be documented and so would be the sensitivity of the test. This however brings up the second problem: patients that are referred to the colonoscopy clinic are not representative of the population at large that are the candidates for mass screening. Indeed, they are at a high risk of developing colorectal cancer. Thus, given the multistep nature of cancer formation and the fact that the biochemical markers are expressed during cancer formation (even before a morphologically visible tumor can be recognized), a good many of these patients are likely to be positive. Be that as it may, we had to do such a study at least to document the sensitivity of the assay.[16,17] In addition to these, studies were also undertaken at Roswell Park Memorial Institute where 10 of 11 cancers were positively identified by the galactose oxidase test (unpublished data).

While this novel concept for early detection of colorectal cancer by examining the rectal mucus and the simple technology for implementing it was greeted with enthusiasm by most, not unexpectedly, a few were skeptical. Quick "studies" were done claiming its 'poor' performance, notwithstanding the fact that the data showed much better performance than the fecal occult blood test (FOBT) and therefore contradicted their own claims.[18] Reports by others, however were much more encouraging. In October, 1989, Sakamoto et al.[19] were the

TABLE 3
Comparison of Galactose Oxidase Test and Hemoccult® Test in
Primary Care Setting[a]

Test	Sensitivity		Negative finding(411)[b]	Specificity
	Cancer (2)	Polyp (14)		
Gal-ox	2 (100%)	11 (79%)	113 (27%)	73%
Hemoccult®	0 (0%)	2 (14%)	37 (9%)	91%

[a] Mean age 58 years, colonoscopy not performed in all cases.
[b] Colonoscopy not performed in all cases.

TABLE 4
Evaluation of Galactose Oxidase Test in Asymptomatic Subject[5]
(Sakamoto Study II)

Test	Sensitivity		Negative finding(294)	Specificity
	Cancer (1)	Polyp (5)		
Gal-ox	1 (100%)	5 (100%)	23 (7.8%)	92.2%
Hemoccult®	0 (0%)	1 (20%)	not adequately evaluated	

TABLE 5
Evaluation of Galactose Oxidase Test in Japan (Kyoto Study)

Diagnosis	Galactose oxidase		Immunological FOBT	
	# of positive/total	(%)	# of positive/total	(%)
Cancer	23/28	(82.1%)	23/28	(82.1%)
Polyp	13/28	(46.4%)	8/28	(28.6%)
Negative endoscopy	7/38	(18.4%)	4/38	(10.5%)

first to report from outside the U.S. on the high performance rate of the test at the Japanese Cancer Association Annual Meeting in Nagoya (Table 2). Sakamoto's study showed that the test not only had a very high sensitivity for colorectal cancer, but that cancers of other organs could also be detected with a fair sensitivity.[20,21] Almost simultaneously in October, 1989, Mackett et al.[22] presented at the American College of Gastroenterology Annual Meeting in New Orleans data on 411 subjects undergoing flexible sigmoidoscopy and other work-ups. Mackett's study also compared the accuracy between the FOBT and the galactose oxidase test. As seen in Table 3, the sensitivity for galactose oxidase in detecting precancerous polyps as well as cancer was far superior to the FOBT. Given the fact that the subjects in Mackett's study were somewhat older, with age ranging from 40 to 83 (average 58) years, not unexpectedly, the specificity of the galactose oxidase test was low (71%). In a second study, Sakamoto et al. addressed this issue in 330 asymptomatic subjects and reported a specificity of 92% in their population[23] (Table 4). Tada et al.,[24] also reporting from Japan, claimed an approximately 82% sensitivity and specificity for the galactose oxidase test (Table 5). While most of these studies were done in high-risk humans in colonoscopy clinics and discovery of cancer or polyp was not unexpected, that by Sakamoto et al.[23] on asymptomatic subjects was the most rewarding for me. I never felt happier than when Ko Sakamoto called me from Japan and told me that he discoverd a cancer in one of the asymptomatic subjects scoring positive (besides several cases with polyps) with the test; I felt that the test has served its purpose and hoped that it (or similar others) would continue to identify cancer and precancer in asymptomatic subjects; my humble effort had been worthwhile.

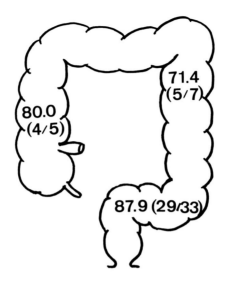

FIGURE 2. Schematic representation of the distribution of the cancers complied from the two studies in Japan.[20,24] Courtesy of Kosaku Sakamoto, M.D., Gunma University School of Medicine, Japan.

TABLE 6
Comparison of Different Tests Recommended for Screening Large Intestinal Cancer

Parameters	Fecal occult blood test	Galactose oxidase test
Sensitivity[a]	4.5–50.0%[25]	80.0–100.0%[12,19]
Specificity[a]	4.3–50.0%[26]	92.2–93.1%[12,23]
Stability	<5 days	>4 years
Restriction	Diet/drug	None
Discomfort	Aesthetic	Minimal
Required #	6	1
Total cost	$8.50	$8.50

[a] For cancer and polyp, the best and worst figures from published reports are given; please refer to specific references for detail.

1. Distribution of Diagnosed Neoplasms

If the field effect theory is indeed the basis of this assay, one would like to see a similar sensitivity for the neoplasms located in the different segments. Figure 2 demonstrates the distribution of 45 cancers compiled from the 2 studies in Japan.[20,24] Commensurate with the field effect theory, the sensitivity is fairly similar for the ascending, transverse, descending, and sigmoid colon and rectum. Table 6 compares the accuracy and costs between the currently popular FOBT and the galactose oxidase test if used for screening large intestinal cancer.

In interpreting these results, I would like to remind readers that there is a great variation in the study design and the study populations, and the end point criteria had also been different. As discussed in Chapter 4, even the so-called gold standard (the colonoscopist's toy) can be less than perfect, depending on the training, experience, and extent of examination of the large intestine. The last fact alone could miss a large number of neoplasms.[27] Thus, further compara-

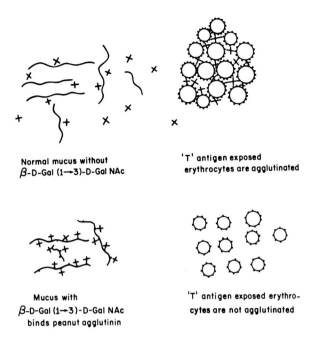

Normal mucus without
β-D-Gal (1→3)-D-Gal NAc

'T' antigen exposed
erythrocytes are agglutinated

Mucus with
β-D-Gal (1→3)-D-Gal NAc
binds peanut agglutinin

'T' antigen exposed erythrocytes are not agglutinated

FIGURE 3. Schematic representation (author's concept) of the principle for hemagglutination inhibition assay. Upper panel: normal mucus glycoprotein (strands) not having recognizable D-Gal-β(1→3)-D-GalNAc fails to bind with PNA (+) which in turn binds with the D-Gal-β(1→3)-D-GalNAc of neuraminidase treated erythrocytes (T antigen) causing agglutination. Lower panel shows cancer or precancerous mucin containing D-Gal-β(1→3)-D-GalNAc (strands with dots) which readily bind with PNA. At optimal PNA concentration, all binding sites will be blocked by the available disaccharide and, therefore, none remaining free for binding with the T antigen on erythrocytes; hence, inhibition of agglutination.

tive studies using proper study population, when done with a clear understanding of the carcinogenesis of colon, would make valid comparisons. In addition, commercial kits would include quality control measures to reduce batch-to-batch variability of galactose oxidase and Schiff's reagent. All things considered, the galactose oxidase test has good potential in our strategies for early detection of colorectal cancer.

III. HEMAGGLUTINATION INHIBITION ASSAY

A. PRINCIPLE

The T antigen (T ag or Thomsen-Friedenreich antigen) is found with a terminal sialic acid residue on the membrane of erythrocytes of human ABO types. This sugar residue appears to be the part of a trans-membrane glycoprotein molecule. Following neuraminidase (or sialidase) treatment, the sialic acid is removed, leaving the D-Gal-β(1→3)-D-GalNAc exposed which can now be detected by specific lectins such as peanut agglutinin (PNA).[28] Because of the common presence of D-Gal-β(1→3)-D-GalNAc in both neuraminidase-treated erythrocytes and colonic mucus in cancer or precancer, Glen Jockle and I had exploited their competitive binding with PNA and developed the hemagglutination inhibition assay (Figure 3).

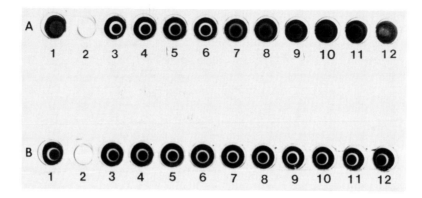

FIGURE 4. Two rows of a 96-well microtiter plate showing hemagglutination inhibition assay are presented. Top row shows control hemagglutination inhibition with serial double concentration of PNA (78 ng.ml⁻¹ in well 3 to 40 µg·ml⁻¹ in wells 1 and 12). Well 1 is positive control for hemagglutination. Note that hemagglutination is inhibited completely in wells 3 through 6, as indicated by the doughnut shaped appearance. Wells 10 through 12 shows agglutination while 7, 8, and 9 show weak inhibition. The bottom row shows a test mucous sample that has inhibited hemagglutination in wells 3 through 12. Well 1 is control hemagglutination inhibition performed by addition of 0.6 *M* ᴅ(+) galactose.

The fundamental principle is still the same one — the field effect theory: the marker sugar ᴅ-Gal-β(1→3)-ᴅ-GalNAc would be present in rectal mucus in patients with cancer or pre-cancer anywhere in the large intestine. Before we started collecting patient samples, we first studied its feasibility by collecting mucus from surgically resected colon of patients with cancer and noncancerous subjects (Table 7). The basic methods of sample colection are pretty much the same as those for galactose oxidase assay.

B. METHODS
1. Collection of Sample

1. Following routine digital rectal examination, dip the gloved examining finger in a specimen bottle containing 500 µl phosphate buffered saline (PBS pH 7.2) containing 0.05% sodium azide.
2. Rinse the gloved finger with the PBS to allow maximum extraction of mucus from the glove.

2. Assay Procedure

1. Make PNA solution in PBS and serially dilute (1:2) from 40 µg ml⁻¹ to 78 µg ml⁻¹ for control hemagglutination.
2. Add 50 µl of serially diluted PNA in the wells of the horizontal row of a 96-well microtiter plate for control hemagglutination, add 0.6 *M* ᴅ(+)galactose for control inhibition.
3. Place 50 µl of mucus solution in the test wells.
4. Add 50 µl of neuraminidase-treated T antigen activated red blood cell to the control and test wells, and incubate at room temperature for 1 h.
5. Inhibition of agglutination is indicated by a doughnut-shaped appearance of the red blood cells in the wells — therefore, presence of ᴅ-Gal-β(1→3)-ᴅ-GalNAc (positive reaction, Figure 4).

Note that this assay has not undergone any further improvements since its development. I am sure that, in due time, the assay could be modified to render it simpler.

TABLE 7
Hemagglutination Inhibition Assay Results

Method of collection	Diagnosis	Positive/total	% Positive
Direct smear of	Cancer	5/5	100
resected colon	Normal	0/3	0
Rectal smear	Cancer	3/3	100
from patients[a]	Polyp	5/10	50
	Normal	14/42	33

[a] Age range 24–89 years.

C. PERFORMANCE

Only one pilot study had been done with this assay; it was composed of (a) mucus samples taken directly from surgically resected colons and (b) rectal mucus samples from 55 individuals (Table 7).

For the surgically resected colons, the mucus samples were collected from the resection margins (10 to 25 cm from the cancer) to test whether or not the rectal mucus sampling would work. All five mucous samples from cancer cases gave a positive hemagglutination reaction. We had tested the stability of the mucous samples in PBS and found that the samples, when stored at 4°C for up to 3 weeks, showed no appreciable change in hemagglutination inhibition. Thus, it is possible to collect the samples at clinics and doctors's offices, even in remote areas, and ship it to a centralized laboratory for assay. A potential added advantage of the assay is that from the standard hemagglutination inhibition, it would be possible to quantitate the amount of D-Gal-$\beta(1\rightarrow3)$-D-GalNAc in the mucous sample. This would allow future correlation with risk of subsequent malignancy in patients with precancerous lesions (e.g., polyps, inflammatory bowel diseases, etc.) or perhaps prognosis. Future research is certainly warranted in this field.

Subsequent study on the rectal mucus from 55 individuals showed inhibition of agglutination in all the 3 patients with cancer, 5 of 10 patients with polyps, and 14 of 42 patients without known colonic diseases. This rather high false positive rate is discouraging; however, it is possible that an improved assay procedure and larger sample size might alter the outcome and make this assay useful in the future. Alternatively, water-insoluble beads agglutination assay could also be developed which would be similar in principle to the hemagglutination inhibition assay (Chapter 6).

REFERENCES

1. **Shamsuddin, A. M.,** Morphological and Histochemical Studies of the Colonic Epithelium of F-344 Rats Treated with Azoxymethane, Doctoral dissertation, University of Maryland at Baltimore, 1979.
2. **Shamsuddin, A. K. M. and Trump, B. F.,** Colon epithelium. II. *In vivo* studies of colon carcinogenesis. Light microscopic, histochemical, and ultrastructural studies of histogenesis of azoxymethane-induced colon carcinomas in Fischer 344 rats, *J. Natl. Cancer Inst.,* 66, 389, 1981.
3. **Shamsuddin, A. K. M. and Trump, B. F.,** Colon epithelium. III. *In vitro* studies of colon carcinogenesis in Fischer 344 rats. *N*-Methyl-*N'*-nitro-*N*-nitrosoguanidine-induced changes in solon epithelium in explant culture, *J. Natl. Cancer Inst.,* 66, 403, 1981.
4. **Shamsuddin, A. K. M., Weiss, L., Phelps, P. C., and Trump, B. F.,** Colon epithelium. IV. Human colon carcinogenesis. Changes in human colon mucosa adjacent to and remote from carcinomas of the colon, *J. Natl. Cancer Inst.,* 66, 413, 1981.
5. **Filipe, M. I. and Branfoot, A. C.,** Abnormal patterns of mucus secretions in apparently normal mucosa of large intestine with carcinoma, *Cancer,* 34, 282, 1974.

6. **Boland, C. R., Montgomery, C. K., and Kim, Y. S.,** Alteration in colonic mucin occurring with cellular differentiation and malignant transformation, *Proc. Natl. Acad. Sci. U.S.A.,* 79, 2051, 1982.

7. **Cooper, H. S.,** Peanut lectin-binding sites in large bowel carcinoma, *Lab. Invest.,* 47, 383, 1982.

8. **Elsayed, A. M., Jockle, G., and Shamsuddin, A. M.,** Peanut agglutinin as a marker for preneoplastic and neoplastic changes in human and rat colon, *Proc. Am. Assoc. Cancer Res.,* 27, 201, 1986.

9. **Shamsuddin, A. M. and Elsayed, A. M.,** Hemagglutination inhibition assay for detection of large intestinal cancer associated glycoconjugates, *Lab. Invest.,* 56, 72A, 1987

10. **Schulte, B. A. and Spicer, S. S.,** Light microscopic histochemical detection of sugar residues in secretory glycoproteins of rodent and human tracheal glands with lectin-horseradish peroxidase conjugates and the galactose oxidase-Schiff sequence, *J. Histochem. Cytochem.,* 31,391, 1983.

11. **Elsayed, A. M. and Shamsuddin, A.,** Detection of altered glycoconjugate in preneoplastic and neoplastic human large intestinal epithelia by galactose oxidase-Schiff sequence, *Lab. Invest ,* 56, 22A, 1987

12. **Shamsuddin, A. M. and Elsayed, A. M.,** A test for detection of colorectal cancer, *Human Pathol.,* 19, 7, 1988.

13. **Shamsuddin, A. K. M. and Harris, C. C.,** Improved enzyme immunoassays using biotin-avidin enzyme complex, *Arch. Pathol. Lab. Med.,* 107, 514, 1983.

14. **Shamsuddin, A. M., Sinopoli, N. T., Hemminki, K., Boesch, R. R., and Harris, C. C.,** Detection of benzo(a)pyrene-DNA adducts in human white blood cells, *Cancer Res.,* 45, 66, 1985.

15. **Shamsuddin, A. M., Elsayed, A. M., and Jockle, G. A.,** Screening test for large intestinal cancer, U.S. Patent no. 4,857,457, 1989.

16. **Knodell, R. G., Hale, E., Antos. M., Matossian, H., and Shamsuddin, A. K. M.,** A new screening test for detection of colon cancer utilizing neoplasia-associated alterations in rectal mucus, *Gastroenterology,* 94, A230, 1988.

17. **Schreiber, J. B., Knodell, R. G., and Shamsuddin, A. K. M.,** Utilization of alterations in colonic mucus as a screening test for detecting colonic neoplasia, *Am. J. Gastroenterol.,* 83, 1058, 1988.

18. **Nsien, E., Steinberg, W., Albert, M., and Henry, J.,** Abnormal rectal mucus test has poor sensitivity and specificity in detecting colon neoplasia, *Gastroenterology,* 96, A368, 1989.

19. **Sakamoto, K., Nakano, G.-I., and Nagamachi, Y.,** Usefulness of a new test for mass screening of cancer in Japan, *Proc. Jpn. Cancer Assoc.,* 48, 332, 1989

20. **Sakamoto, K., Nakano, G.-I., and Nagamachi, Y.,** A pilot study on the usefulness of a new test for mass screening of colorectal cancer in Japan, *Gastroenterol. Jpn.,* 25, 432, 1990.

21. **Sakamoto K., Nagamachi, Y., and Sugawara, I.,** A new screening method for colorectal cancer as a replacement for the Hemoccult blood test, *Jpn. J. Cancer Clinics,* 36, 865, 1990 (in Japanese).

22. **Mackett, C. W., III, Wilson, C. C., Brna, T. G., and Kirkham, R. D.,** Comparison of galactose oxidase test to Hemoccult in colorectal cancer screening, *Am. J. Gastroenterol.,* 84, 1190, 1989.

23. **Sakamoto, K., Muratami, M., Ogawa, T., and Nagamachi, Y.,** Colon cancer screening by a new test: a prospective study of asymptomatic population, *Proc. Am. Assoc. Cancer Res.,* 32, 168, 1991.

24. **Tada, M., Ohtsuka, H., Iso, A., Shimizu, S., Okamura, M., Aoki, Y., and Kawai, K.,** Screening of colorectal cancer by testing rectal mucus for B-D-Gal(1→3)-D-GalNAc (T-antigen), *J. Kyoto Pref. Univ. Med.,* 99, 681, 1990.

25. **Allison, J. E., Feldman R., and Tekawa, I. S.,** Hemoccult screening in detecting colorectal neoplasm: sensitivity, specificity and predictive value: long-term follow-up in a large group practice setting, *Ann. Intern. Med.,* 112, 328, 1990.

26. **Winchester, D. P., Sylvester, J., and Maher, M. L.,** Risks and benefits of mass screening for colorectal neoplasia with the stool guaiac test, *Ca.,* 33,333, 1983.

27. **Johnson, D. A., Gurney, M. S., Volpe, R., Jones, D. M., Van Ness, M. M., Chobanian, S. J., Alvarez, J., Buck, J., Kooyman, G., and Cattau, E. L., Jr.,** A prospective study of the prevalence of colonic neoplasms in asymptomatic patients with an age-related risk, *Gastroenterology,* 94, A209, 1988.

28. **Lotan, R., Skutelsky, E., Danon, D., and Sharon, N.,** The purification, composition and specificity of anti-T lectin from peanut (*Arachis hypogaea*), *J. Biol. Chem.,* 250, 8518, 1975.

Chapter 6

FUTURE ASSAYS AND DIRECTIONS

I. INTRODUCTION

The directions for future strategies for early detection of colorectal cancer should be based on a clear understanding of the pathogenesis of the disease so as to identify and exploit the markers expressed early during cancer formation. That is not to say that our approach in the past and at present has been irrational or illogical; as has been alluded to in Chapter 3, investigations for reliable markers and their potential for application in early detection assays continues, there simply are not many that are practical or reliable or both. Thus, the vacuum has been filled by assays that are either unreliable or impractical for mass screening. In theory, all the markers that were discussed in Chapter 3 have some potential for use in future screening tests as long as they are consistent markers of precancer and cancer. However, much has to happen between the emergence of a marker in the research laboratory and its use in patients. Let us look at future strategies while trying to follow the current-day dissection of carcinogenic events, keeping in mind that a marker for cancer, unless it is detected very early on prior to the invasive stage, is not likely to alter the outcome. Hence, markers of precancer.

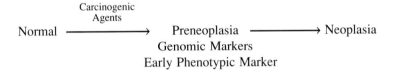

II. ASSAYS FOR GENETIC MARKERS

Since the phenotypic expression of the cell may be controlled by the changes in the gene and cancer cells propagate their altered phenotype to the progeny, the role of the genetic elements in the cell, (DNA, RNA, etc.) in formation of cancer has been an interesting subject. The concept that cancer is the result of alteration in the genetic material is not new.[1] The fact that in the cell the bulk of the genetic material is in the chromosomes, has led investigators to look for alterations there, with rewarding results in some instances (reciprocal translocation between chromosomes as in chronic myelogenous leukemia [Philadelphia chromosome[2]], Burkitt's lymphoma,[3] etc.). The 1980s has seen remarkable excitement in terms of discoveries of the role of genetic elements in cancer, the relatively low prevalence of hereditary cancers notwithstanding, much of which has more to do with the attractiveness of the hypothesis and the weight of the dogma rather than the weight of evidence. In the process, rather hasty extrapolations are being done, most often by the followers of the research rather than the researchers themselves; it is not rare nowadays to hear that the cause of cancer or the cure or both has been found! And colon cancer is not left out in the cold either. Aside from the breakthroughs in the supermarket tabloids, there has been some significant progress in our understanding of the genetic factors in colon cancer, in spite of the rarity of the genetic colon cancers.

A. CYTOGENETIC MARKERS

Familial adenomatous polyposis and Gardner's syndrome are two of the genetic diseases that predispose patients to colon cancer. Herrera et al.[4] demonstrated a deletion on the long arm of chromosome 5 in Gardner's syndrome; linkage analysis established that the gene for familial polyposis is also located on the same chromosome, 5q21-22.[5,6] What, if any, similarity exists between the chromosomal abnormality seen in these familial conditions and in the nonfamilial, sporadic majority? Solomon et al.[7] demonstrated that the alleles at 5q are lost in nearly 20% of patients with nonfamilial colo-rectal carcinomas. Other chromosomes, 1, 17, 18, and 22, are beginning to emerge as important sites for the genetic abnormalities; most commonly, deletions of the short arm of chromosome 17 (17p12 to 17p13.3).[8-13] The region 17p12 to 17p13.3 contains the gene for the protein p53 that plays an important, albeit opposing, roles in transformation. In some experimental systems, it appears to suppress the growth of colon cancer cells *in vitro*.[14]

Undoubtedly these achievements are significant milestones in our learning of the interplay of various factors during cancer formation. What, if any, role they have in carcinogenesis or cancer prevention awaits further work. In terms of their use as markers and practical application in screening, exciting as they may be, they appear impractical. To begin with, the delineation of these changes has to be made by studies of the restriction fragment length polymorphism (RFLP). Polymerase chain reactions, Southern and Northern blot hybridizations, etc. that are labor and time intensive are best carried out in the research laboratory. Even there, at the moment, investigators have considerable difficulty in perfecting the assays and reproducibly performing them, at least at the beginning. Thus, transfer of these technologies for diagnostic purposes will require considerable development, not to speak of their use in mass screening. It is conceivable that these techniques or the simpler and inexpensive surrogates (e.g., immunohistochemical detection of the gene products) could be the assays of the future; but again, to be eligible for diagnosis and screening, their sensitivity of detection has to be better than the current 50%.[15]

B. ALTERED GENE EXPRESSION

From the preceding it is clear that genetic abnormalities are present in about many but not most, much less all, of the cancers of the colon. To summarize, it is now hypothesized that two groups of genes may be important in bringing about the malignant process in the cell: the activated cellular oncogenes and the "tumor suppressor genes". Most of the RNA tumor viruses that causes rather rapid transformation of cells to malignancy contain genetic sequences, called v-*onc* (v for viral and onc for oncogene) which are considered responsible for this action. DNA sequences homologous to many of the v-*onc* have been found in untransformed cells and they are named c-*onc* (for cellular oncogene). Because of the structural homology between the c-*onc* and v-*onc* (albeit much less than 100%), the notion that c-*onc* may have tumorigenic potential became quite attractive despite arguments against it.[16,17] It is presumed that as a part of evolutionary process the acute transforming retroviruses have acquired the *onc* from the "normal" cells during recombination through infection of the host (transduction). Although activated oncogenes could be found in only 10 to 30% of human cancers, it has nevertheless given birth to the hypothesis, popular among many, that activation of cellular oncogene(s) causes cancer. The story becomes even more interesting with the concept of suppressor genes, once considered to be oncogenes, being responsible for cancer.[18] Once again, only after the initial excitement is over, the data and concepts are time-tested, and these marker gene products (oncogenes, suppressor genes, or any other) are documented to be expressed in the majority of colon cancer; they may be used in diagnostic and/or screening assays. In this regard, the DNA ploidy analysis from DNA histogram using flow cytometry appears to be the assay of the nearer future.[19] This technology has the advantage of recognizing the DNA alterations in cells that are yet to show classical morphological features of dysplasia or malignancy.[19-21]

C. CARCINOGEN ADDUCTS

It is the current dogma that carcinogenic agents are responsible for the vast majority of the cancers in humans including that of the large intestine; and the carcinogens are considered to result in cancer formation by binding with DNA. Binding with RNA or other cellular macromolecules have also been demonstrated and detection of these carcinogen-macromolecular adducts may serve as molecular markers of carcinogen exposure and, therefore, susceptibility.[22] Such a strategy is feasible with carcinogens that have been identified and incriminated to particular cancers, such as aflatoxin in hepatocellular carcinoma or benzo[a]pyrene in cigarette smokers and lung cancer.[23,24] However, as regards colon cancer, we are not sure as to the exact chemical carcinogen responsible for the disease, much less its mechanism of action. Recent data from my laboratory have indicated that the fecapentaenes (FP) may be carcinogenic and that putative FP-DNA could be identified *in vitro*.[25] Other DNA damages such as single strand breaks, formation of 8-hydroxydeoxyguanosine by FP has also been recognized.[26,27] The methodologies for their detection are not too complicated, but the science itself has to be further understood; is FP indeed a carcinogen? It would therefore be a while before such approaches will see practical application as assays for early detection of individuals at risk for colon cancer.

III. ASSAYS FOR PHENOTYPIC MARKERS

A. CARBOHYDRATE MARKERS

The carbohydrate markers that appear to have potential application in diagnostic or screening assays in the future are those in the glycoconjugate family, of which the glycoproteins in mucin may be more practical. This may, in part, be due to the fact that mucin is a normal secretion of the large intestinal epithelium that could be sampled in a relatively noninvasive manner. The addition of *N*-acetylgalactosamine (GalNAc, Tn antigen) to a serine or threonine residue may be one of the earliest events in the synthesis of the mucin glycoprotein chain, followed by addition of sialic acid (= Sialosyl Tn antigen), or galactose (= T antigen), or other sugars.[28]

Tn Antigen :	GalNAc—Ser/Thr
T Antigen:	Gal-$\beta(1\rightarrow3)$-GalNAc—Ser/Thr

The concept of field effect change in the entire large intestine in patients with colonic cancer or precancer and the usefulness of T antigen [Gal $\beta(1\rightarrow3)$ GalNAc) as a marker resulting in development of the galactose oxidase and hemagglutination assay has been discussed in Chapters 3 and 5. In brief, the rectal mucus obtained during routine digital examination can be used for detecting qualitative abnormality of the mucin, reflective of the lesion elsewhere in the large intestine. Using the same principle of rectal mucous test and the same marker, my co-workers and I have developed additional assays[29] that could be useful in early detection and prevention of colon cancer.

1. Bead Agglutination Assay for Gal-$\beta(1\rightarrow3)$-GalNAc

The water-insoluble beads such as latex, agarose, etc. can be coated with the lectin derived from *Arachis hypogaea* (peanut agglutinin — PNA) to bind with Gal-$\beta(1\rightarrow3)$-GalNAc (also with Gal, albeit at low affinity). The Gal-$\beta(1\rightarrow3)$-GalNAc (Gal-GalNAc) in the rectal mucous

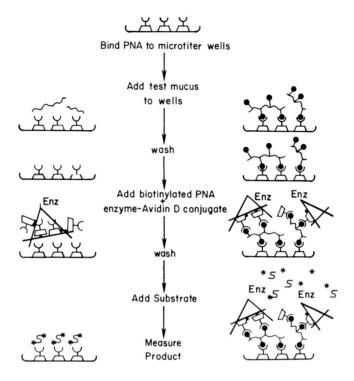

FIGURE 1. Schematic representation of the quantitative enzyme assay for Gal-GalNAc in rectal mucin. The left panel depicts the events in the microtiter well as if the Gal-GalNAc binding site for PNA is masked. Masking of Gal-GalNAc by sialic acid (normal mucin) will cause the solid-phase PNA not to react with the mucin; subsequent washing will remove the mucous glycoprotein (strands) and the biotinylated PNA + avidin-enzyme complex will not bind either, resulting in no enzyme activity and hence no substrate reaction. The right column shows the events if unmasked Gal-GalNAc (pin heads) is present in the mucous glycoprotein sample, allowing it to bind to the solid-phase PNA. At optimum ratio of solid phase PNA and Gal-GalNAc, some Gal-GalNAc sites will remain free, allowing the biotinylated PNA + enzyme-conjugated avidin to bind; washing will not remove the bound Gal-GalNAc and the enzyme resulting in subsequent substrate reaction. By using increasing amounts of Gal-GalNAc, a standard curve can be generated which would allow quantitation of the marker in the unknown sample.

glycoprotein chain of patients with cancer or precancer are likely to bind with PNA coated on the beads, resulting in agglutination; whereas, the Gal-GalNAc in the rectal mucus from normal individuals would be prevented from binding with PNA owing to the attached sialic acid (no agglutination). This is a simple assay that could be acceptable to the public, thanks to the pregnancy tests based on a similar principle of agglutination of insoluble beads.

2. Enzyme Immunoassay for Gal-$\beta(1\rightarrow3)$-GalNAc

The property of PNA to bind with Gal-$\beta(1\rightarrow3)$-GalNAc and the ease at which these lectins can be conjugated with various enzymes and marker substances has resulted in the development of an assay for the determination of this marker carbohydrate moiety. Using the 96-well microtiter assay system (similar to ELISA), it is conceivable that quantitative determination of Gal-$\beta(1\rightarrow3)$-GalNAc (Gal-GalNAc) can be made. In one design (Figure 1), variable but known amounts of PNA is coated in the microtiter wells to render it immobilized onto the solid substrate. Aliquots of rectal mucus dissolved in phosphate buffered saline are added to the wells, followed by a mixture of avidin D – enzyme complex (premixed to yield better sensitivity[30]) + biotinylated PNA. If the sample has PNA-reactive Gal-GalNAc, subsequent washing will not remove the enzyme complex; addition of appropriate substrate for the enzyme will give a color reaction that can be quantitated with a spectrophotometer. The quantity of Gal-GalNAc could be determined by comparing with a standard control.

As opposed to the hemagglutination inhibition, galactose oxidase, or the latex agglutination assay, this enzyme assay offers the possibility of correlating the risk of malignancy with the quantity of Gal-GalNAc present in the mucous glycoprotein. Thus, this test could be of potential use in monitoring people with ulcerative colitis, Crohn's disease, post-resection metachronous lesions, etc.

3. Other Carbohydrate Markers

Via immunocytochemical studies using monoclonal antibodies and lectin binding assay, Itzkowitz et al.[28] have demonstrated the presence of Tn antigen (GalNAc) and sialosyl Tn as oncofetal markers in colon. In a study of 128 colorectal carcinoma specimens, Itzkowitz and co-workers found the expression of sialosyl Tn in 87.5% tumors with a correlation with disease-free and overall 5-year survival.[31] Sialosyl Tn antigen negative tumors had much better prognosis than antigen positive tumors. Thus, monitoring of sialosyl Tn expression could be a useful prognostic indicator.

B. IMMUNOLOGICAL MARKERS

In our quest for identification of malignancies, one group of investigators has pursued the use of immunology in their attempt to identify tumor markers. A variety of antigenic determinants (glycoproteins, glycolipids, or poorly characterized molecules) from cancer cells has served as tumor markers, although very few have proved to be of practical use; keep in mind that because many of these antigens are ill defined, the common practice is referred by the name or number of the antibody. A common approach for obtaining tumor antigens has been to extract the cell surface components from the tissue, which demonstrates that the surface antigens (whatever they may be) of human tumor cells are different from their normal counterpart.[32,33] Because of the presence of this new antigenicity in tumor, it is therefore natural that the normal, otherwise immunocompetent, host would mount a humoral or cellular response, or both, and the presence of circulating immune complexes in the serum of cancer patients has been demontrated,[34-36] However, identification of a specific cancer type may not necessarily be done. Using a capillary culture system to grow human colon cancer cells and a radioimmunoassay, Chester et al.[37] demonstrated that at least half of early stage cancers of the colon (Dukes A and B) could be detected.

Exploitation of these evoked immunity in cancer patients has resulted in the development of other tests such as the leucocyte adherence inhibition (LAI) assay.[38] In short, when leucocytes (monocytes, presumably coated with antitumor antibody) of patients with cancer (early stage colon cancer, Dukes A and B when there is a presumed antibody excess) are incubated with colon tumor extracts, the leucocytes lose their normal ability to adhere to glass.

CD1 (clusters of differentiation 1) molecules are a family of MHC (major histocompatibility complex) class I-like molecules which are expressed on the surface of lymphocytes (immature cortical thymocytes and a subpopulation of B cells), Langerhan cells, and dermal dendritic cells in the human. Five apparently functional CD1 genes are clustered on chromosome 1 (MHC genes are on chromosome 6). The human CD1 locus encodes a family of immunologically different glycoproteins that bind to β_2 microglobulin and CD1 may be important in T cell recognition. Using monoclonal antibody against murine CD1, Bleicher et al.[39] recently demonstrated rather prominent expression of CD1 in murine gastrointestinal epithelial cells, including the colon. At this point, its significance is not clear; it could give some clues regarding the pathogenesis of inflammatory bowel diseases and, conceivably,

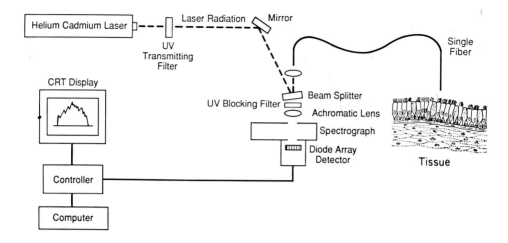

FIGURE 2. Schematic representation of the experimental fiberoptic LIF spectroscopy. (From Kapadia, C. R., Cutruzzola, F. W., O'Brien, K. M., Stetz, M. L., Enriquez, R., and Deckelbaum, L. I., *Gastroenterology*, 99, 150, 1990. With permission.)

along with that an altered pattern of expression could serve as a marker in those conditions which could also be exploited for development of diagnostic assays.

C. LASER-INDUCED FLUORESCENCE SPECTROSCOPY

Utilizing the facts that (1) low-power laser radiation is capable of inducing autofluorescence from tissues without causing damage and (2) laser-induced fluorescence (LIF) spectra between normal and abnormal tissue are different, Kapadia et al.[40] have demonstrated a potential usefulness of this technology in early diagnosis of colorectal neoplasia. In an experimental apparatus, UV radiation from a continuous-wave helium-cadmium laser operating at a wavelength of 325 nm (5 to 10 mW) was coupled to a single 400-μm optical fiber to induce endogenous tissue fluorescence at the colonic tissue site. The induced fluorescence was collected and transmitted by the same optical fiber to a spectrograph (Figure 2). Tissue fluorescence was spectrally dispersed (grating 150 grooves per mm; blaze 450 nm) and imaged onto an intensified diode array detector. The spectrum was plotted on a CRT display and stored and analyzed by a microcomputer. In their pilot study, Kapadia et al.[40] performed fluorescence spectroscopy on polyps (47 adenomatous polyps, and 16 hyperplastic polyps) removed at colonoscopy and on specimens of normal appearing colonic mucosa obtained at colonoscopy or surgery. The shape of the mean spectra are visually different for normal colonic mucosa and the adenomatous polyps. Stepwise multivariate linear regression LIF scores were then plotted for the adenomatous and normal mucosa (Figure 3). The mean LIF scores were $+0.86 \pm 0.06$ for normal colonic mucosa and -0.86 ± 0.06 for adenomatous mucosa ($p < 0.001$). Using an LIF score of $=0.08$ as a cutoff value, the authors report that 100% of the 35 normal and 35 adenomatous specimens could be correctly classified.[40] Undoubtedly this technology has great promise in identifying intraepithelial lesions such as dysplasia or carcinoma in flat nonpolypoid mucosa. We await further development in this field.

IV. INTERVENTION STRATEGIES FOR HIGH-RISK SUBJECTS

At the beginning, I discussed the issue that one of the most important requirements of a screening program is an implied benefit to the participant. As a result of detection of a cancer or precancerous polyp by diagnostic or screening assays, the usual course of action would be

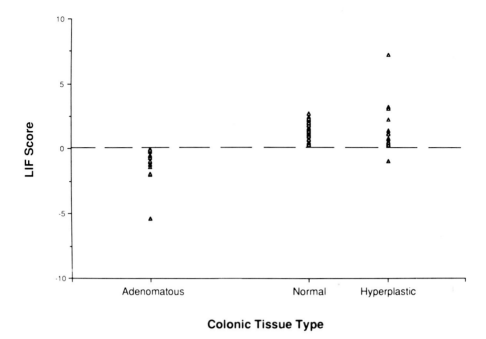

FIGURE 3. Laser-induced fluorescence scores of the normal and adenomatous tissue in the training set. (From Kapadia, C. R., Cutruzzola, F. W., O'Brien, K. M., Stetz, M. L., Enriquez, R., and Deckelbaum, L. I., *Gastroenterology,* 99, 150, 1990. With permission.)

surgical removal of the lesion, the extent of disease permitting; the simple pedunculated polyps can be rather efficiently removed by snare loop polypectomy by the gastroenterologist during endoscopic visualization. However, in many a cases, the lesion will not be detected by the current technology (as discussed in Chapter 2), even with new technologies we might miss. In another example, patients who have undergone resection of the colon for cancer are at a high risk to have metachronous cancer. The current strategy is prevention in these high-risk individuals.

A host of substances have been claimed to have an anticancer effect since time immemorial, but very few have withstood the test of time. For colon cancer, dietary calcium supplementation has been reported to be useful in suppressing the increased cell proliferation in patients with familial polyposis coli.[41] Since then, a plethora of reports have appeared in the literature, both supporting and refuting the beneficial effect of calcium supplementation in experimental systems; a recent study in humans has shown that dietary calcium supplementation over a long term does not reduce the risk for colon cancer, as determined by cell proliferation markers.[42]

While dietary calcium supplementation has been tested on the human, other chemopreventive agents with great promise have only recently been discovered and are yet to undergo clinical trials. Noteworthy are (1) the marine natural product, albeit a rare substance — Sarcophytol, that has been demonstrated to be highly effective in preventing colonic and other cancers in animal models with very little toxicity,[43] and (2) nonsteroidal anti-inflammatory agents (Piroxicam, Sulindac, and difluoromethylornithine).[44,45] My personal effort in this regard has been the anticancer action of inositol and inositol hexaphosphate (InsP$_6$), natural constituents of a cereal diet; to date, they have been reproducibly effective in several experimental systems, yet virtually nontoxic.[46,47] Naturally occurring organosulfur compounds present in garlic and onion oil have also been shown to have chemopreventive function in experimental models and therefore also hold promise for the future.[48]

REFERENCES

1. **Boveri, T.,** Zur Frage der Entstehung Malinger Tumoren, *Fischer,* Jena, Germany, 1914.
2. **Nowell, P. C. and Hungerford, D. A.,** A minute chromosome in human chronic granulocytic leukemia, *Science,* 132, 1497, 1960.
3. **Manolov, G. and Manolova, Y.,** Marker band in one chromosome 14 from Burkitt lymphomas, *Nature (London),* 237, 33, 1972.
4. **Herrera, L., Kakati, S., Givas, L., Pietrzak, E., and Sandberg, A. A.,** Gardner syndrome in a man with an interstitial deletion of 5q, *Am. J. Med. Genet.,* 25, 473, 1986.
5. **Leppert, M., Dobbs, M., Scambler, P., O'Connell, P., Nakamura, Y., Stauffer, D., Woodward, S., Burt, R., Hughes, J., Gardner, E., Lathrop, M., Wasmuth, J., Lalouel, J.-M., and White, R.,** The gene for familial polyposis coli maps to the long arm of chromosome 5, *Science,* 238, 1411, 1987.
6. **Bodmer, W. F., Bailey, C. J., Bodmer, J., Bussey, H. J. R., Ellis, A., Gorman, P., Lucibello, F. C., Murday, V. A., Rider, S. H., Scambler, P., Sheer, D., Solomon, E., and Spurr, N. K.,** Localization of the gene for familial adenomatous polyposis on chromosome 5, *Nature (London),* 328, 614, 1987.
7. **Solomon, E., Voss, R., Hall, V., Bodmer, W. F., Jass, J. R., Jeffreys, A. J., Lucibello, F. C., Patel, I., and Rider, S. H.,** Chromosome 5 allele loss in human colorectal carcinomas, *Nature (London),* 328, 616, 1987.
8. **Reichmann, A., Martin, P., and Levin, B.,** Chromosomal banding patterns in human large bowel cancer, *Int. J. Cancer,* 28, 431, 1981.
9. **Muleris, M., Salmon, R. J., Zafrani, B., Girodet, J., and Dutrillaux, B.,** Consistent deficiencies of chromosome 18 and of the short arm of chromosome 17 in eleven cases of human large bowel cancer: a possible recessive determinism, *Ann. Genet. (Paris),* 28, 206, 1985.
10. **Fearon, E. R., Hamilton, S. R., and Vogelstein, B.,** Clonal analysis of human colorectal tumors, *Science,* 238, 193, 1987.
11. **Fearon, E. R., Cho, K. R., Nigro, J. M., Kern, S. E ., Simons, J. W., Ruppert, J. M., Hamilton, S. R., Priesinger, A. C., Thomas, G., Kinzler, K. W., and Vogelstein, B.,** Identification of a chromosome 18q gene that is altered in colorectal cancers, *Science,* 247, 49, 1990.
12. **Baker, S. J., Fearon, E. R., Nigro, J. M., Hamilton, S. R., Preisinger, A. C., Jessup, J. M., van Tuinen, P., Ledbetter, D. H., Barker, D. F., Nakamura, Y., White, R., and Vogelstein, B.,** Chromosomal 17 deletions and p53 gene mutations in colorectal carcinomas, *Science,* 244, 217, 1989.
13. **Leister, I., Weith, A., Bruderlein, S., Cziepluch C., Kangwanpong, D., Schlag, P., and Schwab, M.,** Human colorectal cancer: high frequency of deletions at chromosome 1p35, *Cancer Res.,* 50, 7232, 1990.
14. **Baker, S. J., Markowitz, S., Fearon, E. R., Willson, J. K. V., and Vogelstein, B.,** Suppression of human colorectal carcinoma cell growth by wild-type p53, *Science,* 249, 912, 1990.
15. **Nigro, J. M., Baker, S. J., Preisinger, A. C., Jessup, J. M., Hostetter, R., Cleary, K., Bigner, S. H., Davidson, N., Baylin, S., Devilee, P., Glover, T., Collins, F. S., Weston, A., Modali, R., Harris, C.C., and Vogelstein, B.,** Mutation in the *p53* gene occur in diverse human tumour types, *Nature (London),* 342, 705, 1989.
16. **Duesberg, P. H.,** Retroviruses as carcinogens and pathogens: expectations and reality, *Cancer Res.,* 47, 1199, 1987.
17. **Duesberg, P. H.,** Activated proto-onc genes: sufficient or necessary for cancer?, *Science,* 228, 669, 1985.
18. **Stanbridge, E. J.,** Identifying tumor suppressor genes in human colorectal cancer, *Science,* 247, 12, 1990.
19. **Ngoi, S. S., Staiano-Coico, L., Godwin, T. A., Wong, R. J., and DeCosse, J. J.,** Abnormal DNA ploidy and proliferative patterns in superficial colonic epithelium adjacent to colorectal cancer, *Cancer,* 66,953, 1990.
20. **Fischbach, W., Mossner, J., Seyschab, H., and Hohn, H.,** Tissue carcinoembryonic antigen and DNA aneuploidy in precancerous and cancerous colorectal lesions, *Cancer,* 65, 1820, 1990.
21. **Kouri, M., Laasonen, A., Mecklin, J.-P., Jarvinen, H., Franssila, K., and Pyrhonen, S.,** Diploid predominance in hereditary nonpolyposis colorectal carcinoma evaluated by flow cytometry, *Cancer,* 65, 1825, 1990.
22. **Harris, C. C., Vahakangas, K., Autrup, H., Trivers, G. E., Shamsuddin, A. K. M., Trump, B. F., Boman, B. M., and Mann, D. L.,** Biochemical and molecular epidemiology of human cancer risk, in *The Pathologist and The Environment,* Scarpelli, D. G., Craighead, J. E., and Kaufman, N., Eds., Williams & Wilkins, Baltimore, 1985, 140.
23. **Shamsuddin, A. K. M., Sinopoli, N. T., Hemminki, K., Boesch, R. R., and Harris, C. C.,** Detection of benzo(a)pyrene-DNA adducts in human white blood cells, *Cancer Res.,* 45, 66, 1985.
24. **Harris, C. C., Vahakangas, K., Newman, M., Trivers, G. E., Shamsuddin, A., Sinopoli, N., Mann, D. L., and Wright, W. E.,** Detection of putative benzo(a)pyrene diolepoxide-DNA adducts in peripheral blood lymphocytes and antibodies to the adducts in sera from coke oven workers, *Proc. Natl. Acad. Sci. U.S.A.,* 82, 6672, 1985.
25. **Shamsuddin, A. M., Ullah, A., Baten, A., and Hale, E.,** Stability of fecapentaene 12 and its carcinogenicity in Fischer 344 rats, *Carcinogenesis,* 12, 601, 1991.

26. **Hinzman, M. J., Novotny, C., Ullah, A., and Shamsuddin, A. M.,** Fecal mutagen fecapentaene-12 damages mammalian colon epithelial DNA, *Carcinogenesis,* 8, 1475, 1987.

27. **Shioya, M., Wakabayashi, K., Yamashita, K., Nagao, M., and Sugimura, T.,** Formation of 8-hydroxyde-oxyguanosine in DNA treated with fecapentaene-12 and -14, *Mut. Res.,* 215, 91, 1989.

28. **Itzkowitz, S. H., Yuan, M., Montgomery, C. R., Kjeldsen, T., Takahasi, H. K., Bigbee, W. L., and Kim, Y. S.,** Expression of Tn, sialosyl Tn, and T antigen in human colon cancer, *Cancer Res.,* 49, 197, 1989.

29. **Shamsuddin, A. M., Elsayed, A. M., and Jockle, G. A.,** Screening test for large intestinal cancer, United States Patent 4,857 457, 1989.

30. **Shamsuddin, A. K. M. and Harris, C. C.,** Improved enzyme immunoassays using biotin-avidin enzyme complex, *Arch. Pathol. Lab. Med.,* 107, 514, 1983.

31. **Itzkowitz, S. H., Bloom, E. J., Kokal, W. A., Modin, G., Hakomori, S.-I., and Kim, Y. S.,** Sialosyl-Tn — a novel mucin antigen associated with prognosis in colorectal cancer patients, *Cancer,* 66, 1960, 1990.

32. **Hellstrom, K. E. and Hellstrom, I.,** Lymphocyte mediated cytotoxicity and blocking serum activity to tumor antigens, *Adv. Immunol.,* 18, 209, 1974.

33. **Hellstrom, I., Hellstrom, K. E., and Sjogren, H. P.,** Demonstration of cell mediated immunity to human neoplasms of various histological types, *Int. J. Cancer,* 7,1, 1972.

34. **Rossen, R. D., Reisberg, M. A., Hersch, E. M., and Gutterman, J. U.,** The C1q binding test for soluble immune complexes: clinical correlations obtained in patients with cancer, *J. Natl. Cancer Inst.,* 58, 1205, 1977.

35. **Teshima, H., Wanebe, H., Pinsky, C., and Day, N. K.,** Circulating immune complexes detected by ^{125}I-C1q deviation test in sera of cancer patients, *J. Clin. Invest.,* 59, 1134, 1977.

36. **Theofilopoulos, A. N., Wilson, C. B., and Dixon, F. J.,** The Raji cell radioimmunoassay for detecting immune complexes in human sera, *J. Clin. Invest.,* 57, 169, 1976.

37. **Chester, S. J., Maimonis, P., Meitner, P. A., and Vezeridis, M. P.,** An analysis of immunecomplexes for the detection of the early stages of colon cancer, *Cancer,* 65,1338, 1990.

38. **Tataryn, D. N., MacFarlane, J. K., Murray, D., and Thompson, D. M. P.,** Tube leucocyte adherence inhibition assay in gastrointestinal cancer, *Cancer,* 43, 898, 1979.

39. **Bleicher, P. A., Balk, S. P., Hagen, S. J., Blumberg, R. S., Flotte, T. J., and Terhorst, C.,** Expression of murine CD1 on gastrointestinal epithelium, *Science,* 250, 679, 1990.

40. **Kapadia, C. R., Cutruzzola, F. W., O'Brien, K. M., Stetz, M. L., Enriquez, R., and Deckelbaum, L. I.,** Laser-induced fluorescence spectroscopy of human colonic mucosa, *Gastroenterology,* 99, 150, 1990.

41. **Lipkin, M. and Newmark, H.,** Effect of added dietary calcium on colonic epithelial cell proliferation in subjects at high risk for familial colon cancer, *N. Engl. J. Med.,* 313, 1381, 1985.

42. **Stern, H. S., Gregoire, R. C., Kashtan, H., Stadler, J., and Bruce, W. R.,** Long-term effects of dietary calcium on the risk markers for colon cancer in patients with familial polyposis, *Surgery,* 108, 528, 1990.

43. **Narisawa, T., Takahashi, S., Niwa, M., Fukaura, Y., and Fujiki, H.,** Inhibition of methylnitrosourea-induced large bowel cancer development by Sarcophytol A, a product from a marine soft coral *Sarcophyton glaucum, Cancer Res.,* 49, 3287, 1989.

44. **Reddy, B. S., Nayini, J., Tokumo, K., Rigotty, J., Zang, E., and Kelloff, G.,** Chemoprevention of colon carcinogenesis by concurrent administration of Piroxicam, a nonsteroidal antiinflammatory drug with D,L-α-difluoromethylornithine, an ornithine decarboxylase inhibitor, in diet, *Cancer Res.,* 50, 2562, 1990.

45. **Friend, W. G.,** Sulindac suppression of colorectal polyps in Gardner's syndrome, *Am. Fam. Phys.,* 41, 891, 1990.

46. **Shamsuddin, A. M., Ullah, A., and Chakravarthy, A. K.,** Inositol and inositol hexaphosphate suppress cell proliferation and tumor formation in CD-1 mice, *Carcinogenesis,* 10, 1461, 1989.

47. **Ullah, A. and Shamsuddin, A. M.,** Dose-dependent inhibition of large intestinal cancer by inositol hex-aphosphate in F-344 rats, *Carcinogenesis,* 11, 2219, 1990.

48. **Sumiyoshi, H. and Wargovich, M. J.,** Chemoprevention of 1,2-dimethylhydrazine-induced colon cancer in mice by naturally occurring organosulfur compounds, *Cancer Res.,* 50, 5084, 1990.

EPILOGUE

I would expect that the readers will communicate with me, preferably in writing, pointing out the errors that I have made and giving me their constructive critique. Hopefully, the next edition(s), if any, will be better. Until then, I would like to conclude by giving my recommendations about what I think are the best approaches to detect cancer of the large intestine at an early stage in asymptomatic individuals.

It is almost impossible not to be biased. I have tried not to be, but this is where I shall be. By definition, the screening test must be rapid, simple, cost effective, accurate, acceptable, and would reward the person partaking of it. I cannot think of a simpler test than the routine digital rectal examination that costs no money at all. This procedure has been recommended and continues to be recommended by every clinician, at least in books of clinical practice (although, in real life, the attending physician defers it to the house staff, or the nurse!). Since a good many cancers of the large intestine are within the reach of the examining finger, it should be a mandatory examination, as mandatory as taking the pulse and blood pressure of the patient. Besides cancer of the rectum, the carefully examining finger may also detect abnormalities of the adjacent organs such as the prostate, vagina, uterus, etc.

During the process of a thorough digital rectal examination, the rectal mucus is almost always caught in the glove, a simple smearing of the mucus on the filter paper for the mucus test can be automatic. The high sensitivity and specificity, the low cost, and the simplicity of the mucus test should make it a natural second step following the rectal examination. How often must we do the mucus test? This should be performed as often as the rectal examination, which in turn should be done as an integral part of the physical examination which should be at least once, if not twice a year.

In the event the mucus test is positive, the physician should best decide what additional confirmatory test is to be done since the subsequent steps may be (1) expensive, (2) uncomfortable, and/or (3) confirmatory of a cancer or precancer, a fact the patients often dread to face or accept. The obvious second step procedures are the barium enema and/or complete colonoscopy, followed by the third step procedure of histopathological examination of any suspicious lesion. In the event the mucus test is positive, but the second and third step examinations are unyielding of any visible mass lesions, the patient is still to undergo periodic routine examination and mucus test twice a year, and the second-level examinations are to be performed at the discretion of the physician since many cancers of the large intestine may be microscopic and not be detected by any of these procedures. The physician may at this time wish to prescribe the chemopreventive agents and check for conversion of the test from positive to negative.

Pending future studies with convincing evidence that the screening tests have excellent predictive value, I am currently supportive of the use of radiologic or endoscopic examinations for screening of asymptomatic individuals with a negative test who are known to have a high risk. A good approach would be to combine two or more first-level screening tests should that be necessary for reasons enumerated above.

At what age should we start screening? While cancers of the large intestine have a peak incidence around age 55 to 60 years, most data suggest that it takes 10 to 15 years for the precancerous polyps to become cancer. Coupled with that is the fact that there are many case reports of cancers of the large intestine that have been discovered at ages 30 to 35. Thus I would recommend that we look for this menace as early as 35 years of age.

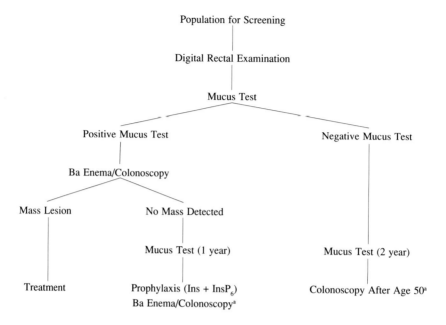

Population for Screening

Digital Rectal Examination

Mucus Test

Positive Mucus Test   Negative Mucus Test

Ba Enema/Colonoscopy

Mass Lesion   No Mass Detected

Mucus Test (1 year)   Mucus Test (2 year)

Treatment   Prophylaxis (Ins + InsP$_6$)   Colonoscopy After Age 50[a]

Ba Enema/Colonoscopy[a]

[a] To be performed at the discretion of the primary physician depending on the merit of the individual cases.

Summary of Shamsuddin's Recommendation (Figure 1):

1. Every individual over the age of 35 years should have a routine digital rectal examination (as a part of a yearly physical examination), followed by mucus test
2. In the event the mucus test is negative on initial examination, it is to be repeated once a year until the age 40; thereafter, twice a year, followed by colonoscopy once every 2 to 3 years beginning at age 50

INDEX